About the ⌐ |

John Brian Ford is a Marriage and Family Therapist licensed to practice in the state of California, USA. He has extensive training in meditative disciplines such as the modern Japanese budo, aikido, in which he holds the teaching rank of 4th Dan, Buddhist meditation practises, and chakra centred yoga. His work as a psychotherapist includes Auto Process Therapy, mindfulness-based therapeutic approaches for stress management, and emotional skill-building to Native American men who are in early substance abuse recovery.

He has worked extensively with populations having severe mental illness in an inpatient setting and at a level fourteen group home. In addition to having a Master's degree in Counselling Psychology, he is an artist and a writer. He currently lives in Sacramento, California with his partner and co-founder of enlightenupyourday.com, a self-paced online therapeutic resource, Theresa Fluty.

Windsor and Maidenhead

9580000194735

Dedication

Dedicated to the courageous men in recovery at Native Directions (Three Rivers Lodge) in Manteca, California. Your insights, humour, commitment, and wisdom have helped greatly in the development of Auto Process Therapy.

John Brian Ford

AUTO PROCESS THERAPY: A THERAPEUTIC APPLICATION OF BUDDHIST PSYCHOLOGY

Revised, Expanded Edition

AUSTIN MACAULEY PUBLISHERS™

LONDON • CAMBRIDGE • NEW YORK • SHARJAH

A CIP catalogue record for this title is available from the British Library.

ISBN 9781787102965 (Paperback)
ISBN 9781528952439 (ePub e-Book)

www.austinmacauley.com

First Published 2021
Austin Macauley Publishers Ltd
1 Canada Square,
Canary Wharf,
London,
E14 5AA

Acknowledgments

There are many people who have been of great support in the writing of Auto Process Therapy; mainly those poor individuals who had to indulge my enthusiastic rants about Auto Process Therapy at odd hours of the morning, afternoon, or evening. I suppose in this sense I have been like a woman expecting a child. I have assumed that everyone around me was as invested in bringing this child to term as I was. And like the friends and family of this hypothetical expecting mother-to-be, the people around me were polite and supportive. For that I thank you! Writing a book is no easy task and requires both gentle criticism and a fair amount of cheerleading from those people who must endure the struggles of the writer. These people include my life partner Theresa Fluty, my siblings, Elaine Smartt, Chris Ford, and my late brother Bruce Ford, who patiently listened to my unsolicited lectures on the relationship between Buddhism and psychotherapy; my fellow MFT and friend, Carlos Oliveira, who offered feedback for, with great interest and zeal, several drafts of the book in its developmental stage, and to my many teachers over the years, both in the field of psychotherapy and Buddhism. To this list of teachers I would include John Smartt, my aikido teacher for over twenty years; the late Tri Thong Dang Sensei who always reminded me to "cultivate equanimity"; the monks at Middlebar Soto Zen Buddhist monastery in Stockton, California; and the many professors of psychology who inspired me in my academic career. Lastly, I must credit my friend and editor, Mira Michele Livingston, with whom I spent many a "hard skull session" refining and revising the contents of this book.

Contents

Foreword *13*

An Overview of Auto Process Therapy *15*

   Key Concepts 15

   Therapy Goals 16

   View of maladaptive behavior 16

   Goals and interventions 16

   Populations 17

   Family Therapy 18

Part One *19*

   Suffering and Liberation 19

Chapter One *21*

   Samsara 21

   Before You Read On 28

Chapter Two *29*

   Object-Self and Process-Self 29

   The Layperson's Perspective 29

   The Clinical Perspective 34

Chapter Three *41*

   Suffering 41

   The Layperson's Perspective 41

   The Clinical Perspective 47

Chapter Four *55*

   The Path of Liberation 55

   The Layperson's Perspective 55

The Clinical Perspective..57

APT Stages of Therapy: Recognition, Acceptance, Hope, and
Treatment...63

Part Two...*65*

Auto Process Therapy: Therapeutic Maneuvers And Stages of
Therapy 65

Chapter Five *67*

Stages of Auto Process Therapy and APT Therapeutic Maneuvers ...67

The Layperson's Perspective 67

The Clinical Perspective..70

Stages of Auto Process Therapy 72

APT Therapeutic Maneuvers 73

Chapter Six..*81*

The Cross Dialectic 81

The Layperson's Perspective 81

The Clinical Perspective..83

Chapter Seven *90*

The Meta-cognitive Reprocessing Maneuver..................90

The Layperson's Perspective 90

The Clinical Perspective..93

Chapter Eight *101*

The Four Behavioral Skills Modules and The APT Diary Card..........101

The Layperson's Perspective 101

The Clinical Perspective..105

The Discernment Skills (Prajna, Right Views)............................ 107
The Ethical Action/Karma Skills (Right Behaviors) 108
Insight Skills (Samadhi, Right Mindfulness).............................. 108
The Compassion Skills (Bodichitta, Right Feelings) 109
Coping Skills Key... 110
The Discernment/Thinking Skills 110
(Accurate Understanding, Wise Views)...................................... 110
The Ethical Action/Behavioral Skills 115

The Insight Skills (Wise Concentration; Mindfulness) 120
The Compassion, Kindness, and Emotion Skills........................ 128
(Heart-Mind) 128

Chapter Nine *142*

Individual Therapy 142

The Layperson's Perspective 142

The Clinical Perspective...147

Chapter Ten.. *157*

A General Overview of APT Group Therapy 157

The Layperson's Perspective 157

The Clinical Perspective...160

Part Three *163*

Addendum Beyond Process Self 163

Chapter Eleven *165*

Towards a Therapeutic Path to Enlightenment.......................165

Developing Calm Abiding 167

Developing Compassion and Loving Kindness.........................171

Direct Perception of Emptiness 173

Meditation on Emptiness 175

Combining the Mental Factors of Enlightenment in Everyday Life .176

Conclusion... *178*

The Future of Auto Process Therapy..178

Glossary of Buddhist and Auto Process Therapy Terms........... *181*

Appendix... *183*

Buddhist Trifecta of Suffering *185*

Buddhist Trifecta of Liberation *186*

The Five Skandhas *187*

Working with Internal Objects... *188*

Behavior and Feeling... *189*

Object-Self versus Process-Self Perspective..............................*190*

The Four Behavioral Coping Skills Modules............................*191*

The Cycle of Cognition *192*

References..*193*

Foreword

Auto Process Therapy (APT) is both the culmination, and the beginning of, a journey I began when I was a fourteen year old adolescent. I suppose you can say that I am the product of the counterculture movement of the 1960s. Born September 2, 1958, I am old enough to remember the "invasion" of the Beatles and the assassinations of President John Kennedy, his brother Robert, and Martin Luther King Jr. I remember the local Catholic priest letting us out of mass early so that we could go home and watch the first moon landing. I worried over the very real prospect of my older brother being drafted into the war in Vietnam. And I hovered around the edges of the many parties my brother hosted as he and his friends learned to play protest songs, experiment with drugs, and grow out their hair.

I am of Irish-American heritage, a practicing Catholic, and a Democrat from a long line of Irish-American Democrats. I still hold to the somewhat romantic notion of a unionized work force and the dream of the Great Society. I grew up in a time when the civil rights movement was just gaining ground and the thought of an African-American president was a far off dream. The fact that I somehow, as an adolescent, found the Dharma of Buddhism at the same time that I discovered Freud is something that I can only call karma.

Like many who feel called to live for a higher purpose my inspiration started with an epiphany. I can clearly remember sitting on the couch gazing into a red glass bottle stopper. It was just a bit of bric-a-brac my mother picked up on one of her trips to the thrift store. Yet within its glass depths I suddenly seemed to perceive the entire universe laid out in microcosm. And it was at that moment that I intuited the existence of a great Truth. That I was unable to articulate the exact nature of this Truth did not deter me one iota from talking about it, with great enthusiasm, to any and all who were indulgent enough to listen. Naturally, I was humored, ignored, and left to my own solitary devices in this matter. Yet, afire with a zealot's determination, I spent hours in the local library and bookstores trying to understand the answer to life's greatest existential questions. It would be many years later that I was able to identify my epiphany as being an intuitive recognition of Buddha Nature.

Over the past forty years I have traveled a long and winding road as I have thrown body and soul into the investigation of reality and the self. My studies have spanned comparative religion, mysticism East and West, aikido, Buddhism, yoga, and psychotherapy. With the formation of APT I have interwoven a lifetime of research and formal education and training into a cohesive, practical Buddhist psychotherapy. APT is neither a mindfulness school of behavioral therapy, nor psychotherapy plus Buddhist thinking. Rather, APT is an original form of Buddhist psychotherapy that is firmly rooted in Buddhism's root premise of no unchanging, abiding self. In place of a self as object, or Object-Self, APT posits the existence of the Process-Self of the moment. From the perspective of the Process-Self we can unhook from the oppressive burden of the Object-Self and the self-recriminations that accompany it. No longer drawn into the depression of the past or the anxieties of the future, instead are we planted firmly in the here-and-now. And it is in this moment that our limitless possibilities are available to us.

I hope this book offers both clinicians and laypeople insights into the true nature of the self, reality, and the possibility of the extinction of suffering. As the Buddha stated many times to his disciples, "By oneself is one rewarded. Work out your salvation with diligence" (Exhortation to the Initiates, Sutra).

An Overview of Auto Process Therapy

Auto Process Therapy (APT) is a psychotherapeutic application of Buddhist psychology. APT is firmly established in the Buddhist theory of no separate, intrinsic self. For this reason APT is an authentic form of Buddhist psychotherapy. Other mindfulness schools of behavioral modification claim an allegiance to Buddhist thinking; APT, by contrast, is predicated entirely upon the Buddha's underlying premise, i.e. that of no actual, intrinsic self-state to be found objectively or subjectively.

Key Concepts

The APT therapist makes four assumptions about the nature of reality: (1) there is no intrinsic self to be found either subjectively or objectively, (2) there is cause and effect or karma, (3) there is re-creation or rebirth of a Process-Self (entire person in-the-moment) from one moment to the next, and (4) there is no reincarnation of an actual self from one lifetime to the next, or, for that matter from one body to the next. In lieu of an intrinsic self, the APT therapist posits the existence of the Process-Self of the moment. The Process-Self, or entire being-in-the-moment, is not an actual self but rather an effect generated continually through the underlying activity of karma. For the purposes of APT, karma is defined as internal, psychological cause and effect driven by choice. The APT therapist views reality as being relational in nature. This is to say, from the standpoint of APT, reality is described as being (1) interconnected, (2) interrelated, and (3) multi-dimensional or "interbeing" in nature (Hanh, p. 244, 2006). Because of the relational nature of reality, the APT therapist holds that no one thing arises independent of other things or conditions. Rather, all things are viewed as being of inter-dependent origination. In Buddhism this state of affairs is referred to as the twelve linked

15

chain of dependent origination. It is the interdependent nature of all things that precludes the existence of a separate, intrinsic self. "The Buddha spoke of the experience of all of this 'mass of suffering' and this suffering comes out of the twelve linked chain of dependent origination". (Noss, 1999, p. 173) Lastly, we suffer because we are in the powerful grip of unconscious attachment to the self-schema. Attachment to the self-schema is the primary delusion from which all other delusions are generated. Delusion gives rise to destructive patterns of thinking, acting, and feeling. Taken together, these three factors (delusion, destructive habits, and negative emotions) interact to produce addiction or grasping, resistance, and denial that constitutes the trifecta of human suffering.

Therapy Goals

The goal of APT is twofold: (1) the moment-to-moment extinction of suffering and (2) to empower the patient to discover their natural equanimity. Equanimity is considered intrinsic to a person's core awareness rather than being a quality that one develops over time. Central to these goals is a profound shift in psychological perspective to that of the Process-Self. Since the Process-Self is only generated one moment at a time, then the extinction of suffering need only occur one moment at a time. Likewise, equanimity need only be realized one moment at a time as well.

View of maladaptive behavior

Maladaptive behavior is seen as the result of attempting to (1) avoid the experience of physical or psychological pain (resistance), (2) grasp that which is seen as providing pleasure (addiction), and (3) ignorance of the selfless, process nature of reality (denial).

Goals and interventions

The primary goals of APT are the extinction of suffering and the realization of a person's (in this case the client's) intrinsic nature of wellbeing. Suffering is defined as being a psychological state of mental anguish and is distinguished from pain. Varying degrees of mental anguish arise when the ego function actively resists the experience of the pain signal. Pain is seen as a natural bioenergetic

16

signal originating in the nervous system that is then interpreted by the mind. As a feedback mechanism, both pain and pleasure inform us as to whether we are in or out of balance. Fear of pain, either of a psychological or physical nature, creates resistance (*dosa*) that then magnifies psychological suffering. Therefore, a central aim of APT is the cultivation of a greatly increased ability to accept the experience of the pain signal. Taken to its logical conclusion this increased ability to accept the pain signal can be defined as unconditional acceptance. Unconditional acceptance has the effect of reducing suffering while increasing psychological balance – even in the continuing presence of the pain feedback signal. Wellbeing is understood to be more than an absence of suffering. Rather, it is an active and dynamic state of ongoing equanimity giving rise to a deep insight into the interdependent and process nature of reality (*sunyata*). The state of psychological equanimity is referred to as *vairagya* in Buddhism. *Vairagya* is a Sanskrit word that is often translated as non-attachment.

Interventions are viewed as therapeutic maneuvers rather than techniques. The APT therapist utilizes a therapeutic process to achieve a shift in psychological orientation. This shift is seen as being away from Object-Self and towards Process-Self. Interventions include a number of meta-cognitive distancing maneuvers such as breath counting, meta-cognitive reprocess or the reprocessing maneuver (RM), guided imagery, and the cross dialectic maneuver. In addition, APT utilizes four essential coping modules consisting of discernment skills *(prajna)*, insight skills (*samadhi*), ethical behavior skills (*karma*), and emotional regulation/compassion skills (*bodichitta*). Mastery of the four APT coping modules is critical to generating a balanced Process-Self. Finally, in order for APT to be its most effective, it is best for the therapist to combine both individual and group therapy from the beginning.

Populations

APT is aligned with positive psychology and therefore best suited for clients who seek to expand on already healthy and adaptive coping behaviors. Nonetheless, other populations who might benefit from APT are individuals with mood disorders, personality disorders, those struggling with chronic pain, substance abuse, post-traumatic stress disorder, and acute stress disorder. Generally speaking, populations under the age of sixteen would not be suitable for APT due to their lack of abstract thinking ability and meta-cognitive development. Those suffering from thought disorders, schizophrenia, and dementia would not be recommended for APT due to poor ego cohesion.

Family Therapy

APT can be applied to the family-as-a-system model by inserting the APT coping modules into the standard framework of family therapy: (1) family goals, (2) positive rules, (3) rewards and consequences, and (4) interventions and strategies. In the case of APT family therapy, the four coping skills modules would be utilized as the basis of the interventions and strategies component of the family systems framework. Additionally, a goal of APT is to achieve a shift in perspective to family-as-process versus the family as an object. This shift will then serve to unhook the individual family members from the family dysfunction. Lastly, such a shift in perspective allows for a refocusing in the direction of the improved quality of the transactions between family members.

Part One
Suffering and Liberation

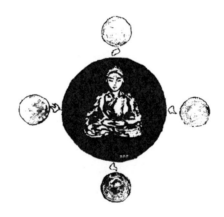

Chapter One
Samsara

*"In every trial let understanding fight for you to defend
what you have won" — The Dhammapada*

*Author's note: The following is my personal account of my descent
into mental illness and substance abuse by which I came to develop
Auto Process Therapy. I believe this story will serve to make the Auto
Process treatment model more meaningful for practitioners and the
layperson; for all too often it is within the context of the struggle for
meaning that wisdom emerges to light our way.*

I came to myself out of darkness floating in a measureless void. It
seemed to me that I was moving forward slowly. I had no sense of
time or place. I was utterly alone in a meaningless universe with only
my fear and pain to keep me company. And then, from somewhere
outside of this realm of nothingness, I began to become aware of
human voices. I could hear my wife talking to my sister. Her words
sent a shockwave of dread through my being, for I cannot say that I
had a body in this state. "If I have to leave Brian to save his life, I
will." Instantly, the full impact of my actions hit me like a blow to
the midsection. I felt shame and horror as I remembered taking a
cocktail of painkillers, muscle relaxers, and alcohol, hoping to end
my suffering once and for all. The events of the past twenty-four
hours came rushing back to me in a flash of memory. I had awakened
to a beautiful day in January. The winds of the previous day had left
the sky clean, blue, and brilliant. Hundreds of people would be living
their lives with happiness and excitement in their hearts. But for me
it was a day of unbearable sadness – for this was the day I decided to
end my life.

I had been struggling with health issues for the past five years. It
began with heart problems leading to a surgical heart valve
replacement. Yet even before the heart surgery I had been slowly

sliding into prescription drug addiction and alcoholism. For me the process of substance addiction was gradual and lacked the dramatic "war story" element so common to the recovery group setting. I had never slept under a bridge or been arrested for public drunkenness. Nonetheless, my addiction had taken its toll on my health, relationships, and career. Making matters worse, I was eight months into a course of medical treatment for a serious illness. The entire ordeal had destroyed my ability to cope emotionally. I was clinically depressed to the point of complete hopelessness. My self-loathing ran so deep that I saw no end in sight to my physical and emotional hell other than to take my own life. I even imagined that I was doing my family and friends a service by doing so. At the same time, at some level I probably wanted to punish a harsh and unfair world for heaping so much misfortune upon me. Had I not tried to be a better person and to help others? Did I not deserve support and encouragement for all of my hard work and sacrifice? Where was the God of mercy and love I had been raised to believe in? Instead, in my mind, I saw only the faces of people looking at me with contempt and scorn. And yet, even after downing my cocktail of painkillers and alcohol I searched through the Bible hoping for a sign. . . for deep inside me the impulse to live was fighting back.

It is a strange function of the mind that we can slip into denial in the face of mortal danger. My denial took the form of housework. In the twenty minutes between taking the pills and passing out on the bathroom floor I began busying myself by cleaning the house. As I returned to the front door after taking the trash to the trashcans outside, I looked up to see a large red-tailed hawk fly only ten feet above the roof of my house. I was struck by the color of its tail feathers that gleamed a brilliant red in the sunlight. I felt overcome by the beauty and wonder of existence. Never had I seen such a thing in all the years I had lived in my home. Maybe there really was a "higher power" at work behind the events of my life. I even considered putting my finger down my throat to rid my body of the poison I had taken. Yet as this internal debate was emerging in my mind the narcotics were taking effect. By the time I reached the bathroom I was losing consciousness. Had it not been for the intervention of my wife, who had come home unexpectedly for lunch, I would have died.

My road to recovery was long and difficult. After agreeing to intensive outpatient therapy, I was released from the hospital and returned home. While in the hospital, I had experienced the worst of the physical withdrawals from the narcotics that I had been addicted to for the past two years. Because of my prolonged use of narcotics my body's ability to cope with pain had been eroded dramatically. Even the slightest bump or scratch could send me into agony. Nonetheless, I adhered to the lessons I had begun to learn in my dialectical behavioral therapy (DBT) group such as "Don't make matters worse than they already are," and "It's not about feeling good in a crisis – it's about being good at feeling." Each day I willed myself to get up and get ready for the daily treatment program, using my newly acquired "opposite to emotions" skills. I threw myself into the DBT diary cards and workbook to the point of memorizing the long lists of DBT coping skills and acronyms as quickly as I could. Along with DBT group therapy, in my individual therapy I was introduced to "positive psychology" and guided meditation techniques. I learned Emotionally Focused Tapping (EFT) and other methods of psychological distancing designed as a shortcut for gaining emotional stability. Moreover, I embraced the Twelve Step Alcoholics Anonymous recovery model by attending AA groups and reading AA's Big Book and other recovery literature. I was completely dedicated to the task of rebuilding my fractured psyche and energized to engage my life. Within a few months of my suicide attempt I was preparing to take the notoriously difficult California State Board exams for Marriage and Family Therapists.

On the personal front my challenges were only just beginning. My marriage of twenty-three years was coming to an end. My wife had resolved to start her life over without the burden of an emotionally unstable husband. In addition to this, I had much to do on the "making amendments" front. I had siblings and old friends whose feelings I had hurt. I felt a tremendous need to heal broken relationships and rebuild the trust I had damaged by my suicide attempt. Yet through it all I found hope in the regime of learning and practicing the behavioral coping skills and the insight building process. I returned to the study of aikido, the art of nonviolent self-defense that I had practiced for many years until my health failed five years before. Why I had stopped going to aikido classes just when I could have benefited from them the most now seemed the height of foolishness to me. I also resumed a daily practice of yoga and mindfulness meditation at the start of my day. I embraced exercise, diet, and nutrition. And above all I forced myself to get out of my house and to be involved with other people by going to church, making coffee dates, and attending AA meetings and social functions. For all of my efforts, by the end of the year my marriage was over, I was unemployed, and I would soon be homeless. Fortunately, I was able to take up temporary residence in the monks' quarters at a local Zen Buddhist monastery. Shortly after, I returned to the workforce as a caseworker for a local resource family agency.

In the process of rebuilding my life I was challenged to go deeper into my investigation of Buddhism and psychology. Through this investigation I began to see the possibility of a Buddhist psychotherapeutic model. My studies for the State Marriage and Family Therapist boards propelled me into the analysis of numerous theories of psychotherapy. Day after day I condensed each of these theories down to their root premise and core principles. That led me to realize that I could apply this same method of analysis to the Buddha's theory of suffering and liberation from suffering. I undertook this challenge with great enthusiasm and set about to write a thesis of Buddhist psychotherapy. Soon I realized that I had the makings of a treatment model for an original form of psychotherapeutic Buddhism.

I continued to practice the skill-building and insight practices that I was developing out of my own journey as a patient. Over time I began to weave them into what would become Auto Process Therapy. One of my first tasks was to apply Marsha Linehan's idea of daily behavior skills coping cards to the Noble Eightfold Path of Buddhism. It became clear to me that Doctor Linehan must have derived her DBT skills modules from Buddhism's Noble Eightfold Path. Applying cognitive behavioral theory to the Noble Eightfold Path, and to Buddhism's "Four Noble Truths" in general, seemed like the obvious starting point. However, because the Eastern approach to "skillful means" does not include much in the way of direct discussion of emotional regulation, I decided to include a "*bodichitta*" or wise heart module.

The Sanskrit word, *chitta*, is often translated as mind. However, *chitta* can also refer to the heart or essence of a thing. *Bodhi* is generally translated as wisdom. With regard to my use of the word *bodichitta* to define a category of emotional regulation, my intention was to approach emotions from an integrative perspective. This is to say, a patient would begin with a simple recognition and acceptance of the emotional experience leading to a deeper understanding of the

Process-Self. (I coined the term, Process-Self as a way to describe a profound shift in experiential perspective). To this end I applied the *bodhicitta* skills to my own often challenging, and still raw, emotional reactions. Needless to say, in this course of self-experimentation life afforded me ample opportunities for practice. Often the simple act of getting out of bed in the morning challenged me to use "paradoxical intentionality" and "unconditional acceptance" to move through the physical pain I felt as my body repaired the damage inflicted upon it by prolonged prescription drug use. An unfortunate side effect of painkillers it that the body loses its natural ability to suppress pain signals. It would be almost a year before my body could tolerate even a moderate amount of physical stress without flooding my brain with agony. It was during this period that I learned to relax and ride the ebb and flow of pain signals. I can remember a feeling like a dagger had raked my legs the day after a challenging aikido class. It was all I could do to expand into the sensation while mentally reframing the pain as feedback or employing Zen Buddhist breath counting methods to create psychological distance. I depended on my healthy routine of morning yoga, meditation, prayer, and other coping maneuvers as I tackled the hours of study needed to pass my state boards for my Marriage Family Therapist license. All the while I wrote down my ideas for Auto Process Therapy until I felt confident that I had something new to offer. By the end of 2014 I had self-published a rough version of Auto Process Therapy: Treatment Model and Practice and had certified one person, "Mary", as a "Life Enhancement Coach". As it turns out, Mary would become instrumental in the editing and refining of APT as a working treatment model. She pushed me to expand on the concepts in the book and would serve as the first person to go through the Reprocessing Maneuver.

In time I began using the emotional skill-building diary cards to help with individual and group counseling. My first significant success would come when working with Native American men at a drug and alcohol recovery program. The site was located on land considered sacred by Native Americans. My relationship with the recovery center had stemmed from my work there as a substance abuse counselor a few years before. I was well aware of the resentment and suspicion many Native men have for white people. Yet, as a recovering person myself, I also understood better than most the challenges of a lifelong, day-to-day struggle to maintain sobriety in a drug saturated society. I appreciated from firsthand experience how reliance on drugs and alcohol can rob a person of basic behavioral coping skills. So it was that I began a weekly APT mindfulness, skill-building group (MSB) with the men in the program. Later I would develop a more intensive, Native Pathways to Recovery group for those men who had graduated from the MSB group.

In retrospect, it was to be expected that I was not greeted with open arms. Even after explaining my history with the center and something of my own struggles in recovery, many of the men nonetheless saw me as a bookish "expert". As such, how could I possibly understand the experience of being a Native man in recovery? Yet through persistent effort I was able to argue the benefits of the skill-building APT diary cards on their own merit. A turning point came when the men collectively grasped the power of linking their behaviors to their feelings. As we sat outside the ceremonial sweat lodge each of the men explained how they were using the coping skills in their daily lives. One man described using the mindfulness skills when playing a game of horseshoes. He became aware of how much damage the drugs had done to his nervous system. Where before he had a command of his mind-body connection, now he had trouble willing his body to obey his mind. But because of his "notice" and "be present" skills he become aware of his condition. Others in the group described finding the positive elements of toxic emotions by using the skill of Accelerated Emotional Integration. In the coming weeks and months the men would find ways to integrate the APT behavioral coping skills to their Twelve Step recovery work in Alcoholics Anonymous. They would share their own discoveries of mindfulness, emotional regulation, insight, and discernment building in group discussions that made mastery of these skills real and relevant to their lives as Native Americans. I was quick to tie these discoveries back into the Native American medicine wheel model of balance and healing. APT, in the beginning, had been just another group to attend in the course of the recovery program; but soon it developed into a way to expand and refine the Alcoholics Anonymous step work and the Native American Wellbriety program. Adopting a truism from Linehan's Dialectical Behavioral Therapy, and combining it with Alcoholics Anonymous' famous Serenity Prayer, I introduced the men to the idea that *serenity* is NOT feeling good; rather, serenity is being able to remain in a state of non-attachment even when one is experiencing distressing feelings. From this perspective we explored serenity as being a feeling that is rooted in a *point-of-view*. Furthermore, I was able to utilize serenity – a central theme of most drug and alcohol recovery programs – as a way to emphasize the role of coping behaviors in the regulation of feeling.

In time I would integrate elements of APT in my work teaching parents strategies to reduce stress and reactivity. I would also bring elements of the emotional skill-building into my individual work with emotionally disturbed children. Again and again I would see the potential of APT to empower clients to greater happiness and peace. And in my own life APT would provide me with a firm foundation to confront my own fears and doubts. So it was that I set out to return, from the standpoint of meditation, to my darkest moment – the place that set in motion the events that would give rise to Auto Process Therapy.

In deep meditation I drifted once again in a dark and limitless void. In this space I had no sense of a time or place. I was utterly alone in an empty and meaningless universe with only my fear and pain to keep me company. I could sense malevolent shapes circling beneath me like obsidian sharks in black water. They waited for me to fall. I saw my past, like a corridor of light, opening to my left. On my right another passage opened to my future. It was bright and warm; and filled with love and hope. And yet, as I floated in the void of suffering, I was acutely aware that this future, and all that might have been, was lost to me forever. Now, however, as I sat in meditation, I proceeded through the stages of the Reprocessing Maneuver.

I am centered in the here-and-now. I reduce my terror to a single statement – I am alone in life. This is a fact. No one will, or can, live my life for me. No one will step in and solve my problems. Like everyone else on this planet I am completely responsible for my own choices. I reflect on the meaning of this truth. If I am alone then I am vulnerable. If I am vulnerable then I will die; I will be nothing. I take a mental step backwards and reduce the thought to a manageable statement – I am a person who is thinking the thought that "I am alone and vulnerable". I notice the emotional charge associated with the thought and I begin to feel fear and doubt. However, before I can become emotionally flooded I shift into a detached state of observation. It is from here, in my detached state, that I can assign color, shape, and texture to my thoughts and feelings. They exist as mere mental objects; or like interesting features of a landscape that I am soaring above. Now, seen from a perspective of detachment, they lose all of their emotional charge. I can understand how the thoughts give rise to the feelings and, in their turn, how the feelings empower thoughts. They exist as mental formations of my own creation. I am aware of my underlying belief in helplessness. It is an old belief that is rooted in my child-ego's misunderstanding of a big and unpredictable world. Behind it all I see the delusion of the Object-Self to which I am fettered. I let go of it and I shift once again; but this time from detachment into non-attachment. My thoughts and feelings flow through me like a stream of clear water. I become one with the moment, and in doing so, I cross into the Process-Self. The darkness of the void becomes the fullness of the universe. In my mind I imagine stars and galaxies filling the empty blackness of space. From the deep place of core awareness a wordless voice rises into my mind: "I am the gateless gate; the one gate that is many. I am suchness." I take a breath and return to myself sitting on my meditation cushion. I ring the bronze Tibetan prayer bell in front of me and stretch. It is a beautiful morning in January. The sky is clean, blue, and brilliant. All throughout the world billions of people are living their lives in happiness, love, and peace. I relax, smile, and breathe. It is a fine day, and I am grateful to be counted among them.

Before You Read On . . .

After self-publishing a rough version of Auto Process Therapy and receiving feedback from fellow mental healthcare professionals as well as laypeople, it became clear to me that many of the ideas and concepts in this book require further explanation in order to be accessible to a broader audience. To this end I have included The Layperson's Perspective at the beginning of each chapter starting with chapter two through chapter ten. In this way I hope that the book's technical information will be more accessible to those readers who are unfamiliar Buddhist tenets and terminology.

Chapter Two
Object-Self and Process-Self

"The 'I AM' is not an entity behind the attributes;
[Rather] it originates by their cooperation" –
Buddha; Exhortation to the Initiates, Sutra

The Layperson's Perspective

From our earliest moments in life we are provided with a picture of ourselves as being separate and alone in an unpredictable universe. Beginning in infancy our parents, educators, political and religious institutions continually bombard us with messages of separation and duality. Yet, upon closer examination, nothing can be further from the truth. Our actual nature is that of pure and free flowing eminence or *beingness* that cannot be pinned down by labels or judgments. Our thoughts and feelings are little more than passing patterns of energy that are driven and sustained by attachment to our unconscious, habitual beliefs, and deeply rooted misconceptions. The greatest misconception of all is that of the separate self-entity or inner person behind our thoughts and feelings. Throughout our lives we strive to change, inflate, or escape this person within – but to no avail. For if such an inner person existed it would have total power over the thinking and feeling processes of the mind. Yet, try as we might, we continually fail to command ourselves to be happy or to control our thoughts at will. The best we can arrive at is to construct a façade of a self with which we can live. We call this façade our self-image. In time, through the power of attachment, our self-image takes on a reality of its own. Our impulse to grasp becomes, "I'm the kind of person who likes this." Our impulse to resist becomes, "I'm the kind of person who doesn't like that." Our lack of awareness becomes, "I'm the kind of person who does not care but this." Over the course of our life we become more or less content with this situation. However, because of the unstoppable forces of time and impermanence, sooner or later we are forced to confront the fiction of our self-image. As we grow older we begin to lose our youthful attractiveness and physical resilience. Perhaps we have a setback in our career and our financial situation precipitously deteriorates. Maybe our marriage fails or we are faced with ending a long-term relationship. Worst of all, a family member or close friend might pass away unexpectedly and so we must cope with a sudden loss. Now the self-image we have been clinging to so tightly is threatened. It is at this point that we suffer the most.

Many people come to therapy in a state of profound distress due to their attachment to an idea of how they *should* be in the world. More to the point, they are in distress because they feel that they are not measuring up to their ideal self as dictated to them since childhood. Others come to therapy with a sense of not knowing who they are at a core level. They feel lost, believing that they should have an answer to this question. In either case the client is in the grip of a powerful attachment to their idea of self. Many forms of psychotherapy are concerned with helping the client to redefine their idea of self in a positive light. However, from the standpoint of Buddhist psychology, the self is a fiction. Hence, it is impossible to fix the self because it simply does not exist in the first place. Furthermore, it is the attachment to this fictitious self that fuels the engine of the client's suffering. If the client were to see the self as an empty effect it might be possible to become non-attached to it. By non-attaching to their self-notion – what is referred to as the Object-Self in Auto Process Therapy – the client is free to engage the present moment with greater mindfulness and ease. A critical first step in arriving at non-attachment is to understand the nature of the ego and its role in grasping.

The ego as a function of the mind, evolved over millions of years in humans. Our primitive ancestors were able to mentally project themselves into hypothetical future situations. This ability gave them a tremendous advantage over other animals. Yet this same inborn advantage works against us in contemporary society. This is because the ego does not have an off switch. Instead, it grinds away ceaselessly and draws us away from the here-and-now. It is the primary function of the ego to make sense and order out of unrefined sensory data and unconscious instinctive drives. In Buddhist psychology functioning of the ego is referred to as *manas*. It is the job of the ego function to organize perceptual elements into a working model or schema. The schema defines what a thing is and what it isn't. A chair schema is a simple model for all chair-objects that includes non-chairs objects such as a couch or a stool.

We begin to create schemas even as infants. Schemas can also be constructed to describe how others relate to us. This type of schema is a relationship schema that informs our expectations of how other people will treat us. For instance, children who are raised in families where there is emotional and/or physical abuse tend to develop negative relationship schemas. They often become angry or fearful adults who struggle with trust and poor self-esteem. On the other end of the spectrum are those people who were raised in families where love, trust, and consistent parenting strategies were the norm. These people tend to carry a positive schema of the world in their mind. For such people life is a gift that is filled with wonder and exciting possibilities. In either case it is the ego's schema-building function that results in the creation, for better or worse, of the personal fiction or inner narrative.

The personal fiction is the story that we carry around in our mind in which we are the central character. So compelling is our attachment to our personal fiction that it has the power to affect our overall mood in dramatic ways. From the moment we wake up in the morning we are involved in the generation of our personal fiction. It is as if we are playing a movie in our mind in which we are fighting the heroic fight against impossible odds. We may also play the role of victim in our personal fiction. When we play the role of victim we feel self-pity and sadness. When we play the role of the avenging hero we feel inflated and perhaps angry. Sometimes we combine the roles of hero and victim and so become the savior. As the savior we assume the part of the self-sacrificing hero who throws himself under the bus for the sake of others. This version of the personal fiction makes us feel virtuous and morally superior. And so it goes, churning away throughout the day and the night. It is not enough that we spend so much time and energy invested in the fictions on our mobile devices or our home entertainment centers; we must also invest in the movie playing inside our mind twenty-four hours a day. More than anything else, it is our attachment to our personal fiction that diverts our attention from the here-and-now; from mindfulness. In our thoughts we are constantly reciting the mantra, "Here's me doing this; here's me doing that." In place of mindfulness we become forgetful and distracted as we grasp after pleasure and push away pain. Yet by doing so we create a dualistic split between self and others and

31

thereby fall into the realm of suffering and delusion. It is this realm, or state of mind, that is called *samara* in Buddhism. To be sure, there are other factors that play into forgetfulness such as fatigue, chronic stress, or sickness. However, it is the powerful draw of our personal fiction that is our central source of distraction and suffering. In Buddhism the generation of the personal fiction is called *becoming*. "The Buddha had a technical term for this sense of self-identity in a particular world of experience: He called it becoming". (DeGraff, 2012, p.9)

There are some forms of psychotherapy, such as Narrative Therapy, that embrace the personal fiction. In Narrative Therapy the client is asked to tell their story in the safety of the therapeutic setting. Upon revealing their story, the client is asked to re-write their personal fiction to make it more adaptive and positive. In this way the client is taking control of the narrative of their life. And where this may be a valid approach to treatment for many people, it fails to address *tanha* or grasping that is at the root of human suffering. From the standpoint of Buddhist psychology the act of investing in our self-fiction is paramount to throwing gasoline on the fire. As long as the client is attached to the notion of being a separate self-entity, they will forever remain in the grip of a chronic dissatisfaction or *dukkha*. Even if the client should manifest their personal fiction in real life they will find that the experience is temporary. Like all things it will pass quickly away leaving the client in a state of disappointment. And now they must set out to recreate their personal fiction all over again. Or the client will actualize their personal fiction only to discover that it is not as wonderful as they imagined. In any case, the client has made their situation worse by strengthening their attachment to an internal representation of reality. Meanwhile, they are missing out on the experience of their moment-to-moment existence with all of its miraculous possibilities.

Auto Process Therapy offers an alternative perspective on what we experience as a "self". This alternative perspective is what I refer to as a Process-Self perspective. When we are in the Process-Self we feel less of a pull from past memories or worries about a hypothetical future. Our perception of time is of a moment-to-moment nature as when we are immersed in an enjoyable task. We have a sense of ease and flow as well as a feeling of warmth and goodwill. People unconsciously perceive this and respond in kind. Very often we have shifted into a state of process but do not realize it. We might be enjoying a trip to the farmer's market or grocery store. We are in no particular hurry and are excited but calm as we explore the food booths or wander the grocery aisles. There is a vivid quality to everything as if our senses have been sharpened or cleaned. Our emotional state is both calm but energized. And underneath it all is an intuition of a deeper awareness behind the everyday workings of the mind. However, because we are driven by unconscious attachments and habitual patterns of thinking and feeling, we soon lose this intuitive sense of selfless ease. A blaring car horn impacts our hearing and without missing a beat we think, "What a jerk!" A divide opens between "us" and "them" and we experience anger and resentment. But these feelings do not jive with our idealized self-image as a nice person; our becoming. It is at this point, if we apply mindful attention, that we can notice subtle currents of anxiety and mental tension. "If I am not a 'nice person' than who am I?" Rather than explore this feeling we distract ourselves by justifying our anger: "Everyone knows that hitting your horn contributes to noise pollution! People should learn to be more patient. At least I am better than that!" Once again we find ourselves hypnotized by our personal fiction and so have become caught up in the dualistic, Object-Self perspective.

It is important to remember that the Process-Self perspective is not the same as the belief that there is no self at all. This argument is a negation of existence. Instead, the Process-Self is one in which the experience of self is fluid, adaptive, and at one with the moment. It is a shift in our point of view that is more expansive and inclusive than ever before. From this point of view there is plenty of room for the full range of our feelings and thinking patterns. We can engage them and let them go as easily as letting the clear water of a mountain stream run through our fingers. It is as if we, ourselves, have become like a stream of free flowing awareness that shares much in common with a mountain stream. And just as the stream is connected to the runoff and snowpack, so we are connected to the source of our own being. For the purposes of Auto Process Therapy, I will call this source of being core awareness. In core awareness there is non-attachment to both the feeling and idea of a self. For in truth, it is grasping and attachment that generates the dualistic split which results in creation of the Object-Self. Instead, through the healing power of non-attachment and unconditional acceptance, we have the experience of awakening to a state of core awareness. In this awakened state words fail us as we take in the essential features of core awareness. In Buddhism these essential features are described as consisting of infinite intelligence and boundless compassion. Like the silver metal that binds the two opposing sides of a coin together, it is core awareness that unites both the Object-Self and the Process-Self perspectives.

In the coming chapters we will explore the origin of suffering and the nature of liberation from suffering: first from the clinical perspective, and then from the layperson's point of view. I will also describe the therapeutic methods of APT in everyday language. For the therapist I would suggest reading from start to finish. If you are a layperson it might be better to begin with The Layperson's Perspective at the beginning of each chapter and then review the technical reading. However, the choice is up to you.

The Clinical Perspective

All of Buddhist theory concerning suffering, the necessary preconditions of suffering, and the ultimate extinction of suffering, are founded upon Siddhartha Gautama Buddha's root hypothesis that there is no actual, distinct self (Object-Self) to be found. "Finally, as the morning star came into view, his mind opened to the reality that no separate Siddhartha really existed. His desire and suffering vanished along with the illusion of his Self." (Metcalf, 2003, p.18) At first this may seem like an inherently contradicting assertion in that there must be some kind of self or who then is reading these words? And indeed, most forms of psychotherapy assume a subjective self that operates behind the various functions and cognitions of the mind. Sometimes this subjective self is labeled the ego; and other times the authentic self or whole that is greater than the sum of its parts as in gestalt theory. "The main idea of Gestalt is that a gestalt is a whole, a complete, in itself." (Perls, 1973, p. 119) Other Western psychologists who tackled the question of the self includes Carl Jung and Carl Rogers. Jung conceived of the self as the central organizing force in the psyche. But it would be Rogers who first developed the concept of a process self. "Self as an object tends to disappear. The self, at this moment, is this feeling. This is a being in-the-moment, with little self-conscious awareness." (Rogers, 1961, p.147) Rogers developed seven stages of therapy that were designed to lead a client through a process to self-awareness and acceptance.

Of all the early theorists, it was Rogers who came the closest to creating a genuine application of Buddhist psychological principles. But according to Buddhist theory there simply is no self to be found. Furthermore, a careful examination of the self-reveals that it is, at best, an empty effect that is generated one moment at a time. "Ultimately, we see that our sense of self, the personal identity we protect so fervently, is an illusion, for we are a process, a constant flow of physical, emotional, and mental events new each moment." (Gunaratana, 2001, p.197) And it is this very moment-to-moment effect, the self-as-process, who is the active participant that reads these words.

Insofar as the meaning behind our words is often as important as what we actually say, I think it crucial to be clear about my own intentions regarding the "no self" hypothesis. As a practitioner of Buddhism I strive to live my life from a self-as-process (Process-Self) perspective (Appendix, Fig 6). However, for the purposes of the application of APT I only ask that you consider temporarily reframing the Object-Self into a more adaptive Process-Self perspective. The central purpose of doing so is to further the investigation of APT as a helpful therapeutic modality. For in truth it is not possible to practice APT from an Object-Self point of view. This being said, it is not my objective to convert anyone to a particular faith tradition or even to renounce the Object-Self perspective in one's personal life. Therefore, having declared my intention, I now ask you to entertain a few of the advantages presented by the Process-Self perspective.

(1) If there is no actual self to be found, but only a Process-Self, then there is no need to chastise or judge ourselves. The self of the past is already gone, and the potential future self may never come into being. Only past karma, which is best described as unconscious behavioral tendencies driven by choice, remains to influence the present.

(2) If the Process-Self is generated one moment at a time then we have only to extinguish suffering one moment at a time. This is a far easier task than attempting to manage one's entire life (past, present, future) all at once.

(3) If the Process-Self is not fixed and unchangeable, but instead fluid and adaptive, then the very real possibility for growth and change is available to us in any moment.

To be sure, I'm sure some of you readers are thinking, "I know of some clients having antisocial personality disorder who will love this no self, no consequences idea." And if not for the law of cause and effect this possibility would pose a very real danger. But the fundamental nature of any process, be it the Process-Self or any number of other processes found in nature, is a series of changes that are governed by origins and conditions. This being the case, there are inevitable consequences for all of our actions. On an internal, psychological level this state of affairs is defined as karma. "Karma is one of the most important words in Buddhism but is often misunderstood. It refers to the cause and effect in relation to the mind". (Tserling, 2006, p. 35) Therefore there may be no "actual" self to be found but there *is* karma. The self of the moment may decide to drink an entire fifth of whiskey or eat an entire chocolate cake in one sitting. However, there is a great likelihood that the potential future self will suffer the negative karma of doing so.

Returning to the discussion of the self-perspective, we can reflect on the self as being the end result of underlying cause and effect or karma. From the standpoint of karma we can also begin to see how we might create a given self-perspective in any given moment. In this sense the self is like a computer-generated animated image that is the result of the ongoing interaction of hardware and software. Karma can be understood as being the dynamic exchange of energy between the computer's memory, processor, and software applications. In the same way the self is like an animated image generated by the exchange of biological and psychological energy. There is no actual person inhabiting the animated image as it is only an empty effect. However, we can argue that the computer-generated image is real enough as a phenomenon. Thus it follows that the relationship between karma and the self is that the self is a form of karma or ongoing dynamic effect. Furthermore, the self-effect can no more be separated from the energetic exchange from which it emerges than a wave on the ocean can be separated from the ocean. And yet, by shifting our perspective from wave to ocean, so to speak, we have the ability to unhook from the static Object-Self perspective and become the very karma (energetic process) we wish to create in our lives.

Looking to nature, I use the example of a river to illustrate the difference between Object-Self and Process-Self. A river is a flowing manifestation of water linked to the streams and tributaries that, themselves, are the result of mountain runoff caused by a melting snowpack. The snow is the result of precipitation caused by evaporation. Much of this evaporation comes from the ocean into which the river is always flowing. So where, in all of this cause and effect, is the actual river to be found? Can we dip a cup into the river and declare that we now have the actual river held captive in a cup? Can we separate the river-*ness* from the river? The true nature of the river is inseparable from the actual river. In the words of the Buddha, "Heat is different from fire in our thoughts, but you cannot remove heat from fire in reality". (Initiates sutra, 1985, p. 45) So it is with process and self. In Auto Process Therapy there is no actual self to be extracted from selfness process of the moment. As with any process, the self is generated by, sustained by, and driven by cause and effect.

What this looks like in terms of psychotherapy is the clinician leading the client through a course of therapy with a clearly defined beginning, middle, and an end. Therefore, in a general sense the overall goals of Auto Process Therapy must always include: (1) helping the client to make a shift in psychological perspective away from attachment to Object-Self and towards the realization of Process-Self, (2) to help the client to counter grasping (addiction), aversion (resistance) and ignorance (denial) in the service of the moment-to-moment extinction of suffering, and (3) assisting the client to generalize the gains made in therapy into daily life. Such a profound shift in perspective must penetrate to the deepest unconscious levels of being if it is to be meaningful. This demands that the therapist must also have achieved a degree of reorientation from Object-Self to Process-Self themselves. APT does not require a leap of faith but simply a willingness to temporarily reframe, with regard to the APT goals and methods of therapy, one's own understanding of self.

Buddhist psychology conceives of the self as existing because of various physical and psychological factors that combine to generate an overall effect. It is this effect that people consider to be a self. The self-as-effect or Process-Self is philosophically opposed to an Object-Self that supposedly functions behind the cognitions of the mind. According to Buddhism, the factors that combine to generate the self are referred to as the five "*skandhas*". (Noss, 1999, p. 181) The five skandhas are aggregates that are generally described as being: *Consciousness, Thoughts, Volitional Formations (also*

Perceptions), *Feelings*, and *Samskaras* or unconscious, behavioral habits and tendencies (Appendix, Fig 3). *Consciousness* is our most basic, pure awareness and is not considered a self; but rather, it is a universal abstraction. Therefore, consciousness can be described as a hypothetical unit of measurement that exists alongside time, space, matter, and energy. (Goswami, 1995, p. 204) Consciousness can also be thought of as being the act of perception in that consciousness, by its very nature, must always be conscious of something. Consciousness, in this context, is of a relative nature and must be distinguished from core awareness. *Thoughts* refer to intentional thinking or thoughts we purposefully invest in, generate, and maintain. Such thoughts are different from automatic thoughts that arise from the unconscious as a reaction to events in our environment. *Volitional Formations* refers to either physical or abstract demarcations and labels. Volitional Formations arise when one of the five senses makes contact with the environment. The raw sensory data generated by the contact between the senses and the environment is labeled and categorized by the mind to create a representation of reality. They are 'volitional' because we habitually invest in our labels as if they are actual manifestations of the underlying reality that they are intended to represent. Feelings are physical sensations that draw us to, or propel us away, from a given stimulus. Feelings can also be of a neutral or dull nature. Physical intuition is another manifestation of feeling. Feelings, in the Buddhist sense of the word, are distinct from moods and emotions. Moods and emotions are labels that are attached to feelings and therefore belong to the realm of the thinking mind. *Behavioral habits* are deeply embedded behavioral scripts that exist as potential behaviors *(bindus)*. The term *bindu* is a Sanskrit word for a seed that lays dormant in the unconscious mind until activated by our intentions or by a stimulus. "When someone says something unpleasant or hurtful to us, he waters the seed of anger in us. The seed manifests itself in our mind consciousness and becomes a mental formation". (Hanh, 2006, p. 78) *Bindus* are referred to as seeds because they lie dormant in our mind-stream waiting to be activated by our intentions. They act as behavioral potentials that can be quickened to give fruit to the state of delusion or enlightenment.

Ultimately, it is the mind that perceives the various cognitions that are generated within the overall field of consciousness. Taken together, the five senses and the conscious mind constitute six of the eight levels of consciousness in Buddhist psychology. The seventh and eighth levels of consciousness are the ego or *manas* level and the store consciousness or Id. Perceptions give rise to either positive, negative, or neutral impulses that in turn prompt behaviors. Behaviors determine feelings that then influence that which we choose to pay attention to and how we prioritize, unconsciously, the importance of what we perceive, i.e., cognitive bias for or against a given experience (Gunaratana, 2001). This overall process can be thought of as cyclical in nature, starting with perception and, ultimately, returning to perception (Appendix, Fig 8).

With regard to the *skandhas*, APT interprets them as consisting of seven coexisting domains that combine to generate the moment-to-moment Process-Self. The seven domains according to APT are the overall field of consciousness that is roughly divided into conscious awareness, the pre-conscious mind, the subconscious mind, the unconscious mind, the collective or socio-cultural unconscious, and lastly core awareness or "the ground of all being". (Goswami, 1995, p. 106) Coexistent with the factor of consciousness are behavioral habits, cognitions, feelings, physical form (the body including genetic predispositions), personality, and the ego function, consisting of what neurologist James Austin referred to as the I-me-mine complex (2001, p.44).

There is much more to be said about the APT perspective on self and suffering. For now, however, it is enough to tackle the root hypothesis upon which APT theory and practice is established. Essential to the APT approach is that there is no unchanging intrinsic self, either objectively or subjectively, to be found. Therefore, attachment to the Object-Self gives rise to the state of psychological anguish or suffering. This being said, the Object-Self is not the enemy. Rather, it is only one side of the coin. In truth, if a human being is to function at their maximum capacity it is necessary to integrate both perspectives – that of the Object-Self and the Process-Self. Only by embracing both perspectives can the client arrive at a more balanced worldview. From this worldview – in which the Object and Process perspectives are held in mind in equal measures – the process nature of a given object is understood on an intuitive and practical level. Simultaneously, from this integrated perspective the object nature is also comprehended on both a feeling and conventional level. To quote from the Buddhist Heart Sutra, "Form is emptiness. Emptiness is form. Indeed they are not different, they are the same". (Tenzin Gyatso, 2005, pp. 144-121) Another way to think of the integration of the Object- and Process-Self perspective is that a given form has the underlying nature of process; and, at the same time all process manifests – in one way or the other – as form.

In the following chapters I will discuss the stages of APT therapy, its goals and interventions, and the relationship of APT group and individual therapy. To those who are unfamiliar with Buddhist thinking and practices many of the concepts in this book may seem alien and difficult to understand at first blush. Nonetheless, the therapeutic value inherent in the Four Noble Truths of Buddhism, upon which APT is directly extrapolated, speaks for itself. For now I only ask that you, the reader, hold an open mind and a willing heart to the possibilities offered by Auto Process Therapy.

Chapter Three
Suffering

*"People are in bondage because they have
not yet removed the idea of ego" –
Buddha; Exhortation to the Initiates, Sutra*

The Layperson's Perspective

Pain and suffering are often lumped together but in reality they are two different things. Pain is nothing more than the body-mind's feedback system warning us that something is out of balance. The purpose of pain is to point us back in the direction of balance. As feedback pain can be either physical or psychological in nature. Physical pain can be of the nerve burning sort or a deep ache. It can also manifest as sharp, hot, cold, throbbing, or as nausea. Psychological pain takes the form of afflictive emotions such as anger, frustration, boredom, fear, or anxiety. Suffering, on the other hand, is defined in Buddhism as ranging on a scale from mile dissatisfaction to intense anguish. The essence of suffering is grasping. We grasp at the fleeting sensation of pleasure. We also grasp at *not* feeling physical and emotional pain. More than anything we grasp at a fixed and separate self-identity that, upon close examination, simply does not exist.

Most people assume that a certain amount of suffering is inevitable in life. We take it for granted that sooner or later we will be faced with painful experiences. Sometimes we accept the suffering that we create for the sake of a short term gain. We might drink too much wine or beer on a Friday night knowing that we will have to contend with a hangover the next morning. We stay up too late trying to finish the last pages of a mystery novel and knowingly sacrifice sleep in the process. We order the extra spicy sauce regardless of the heartburn we know will keep us up the rest of the night. For the most part we try not to think about suffering until it confronts us directly. We whistle past the graveyard, so to speak, rather than consider the inescapable facts of old age, sickness, and death. To this end we engage in the endless pursuit of pleasure while pushing away painful stimuli. We distract ourselves with hours of television, movies, video games, and Internet surfing. In some cases we turn to drugs, alcohol, and reckless adventure seeking. Our grasping can take the form of striving for the perfect partner in life. We might spend hours on Internet dating sites or making the rounds of the pickup bars and clubs. This can lead to a string of broken relationships or irresponsible and dangerous sexual encounters. We seek to acquire more and more material possessions that never seem to fill the void in our hearts. Driving all of this is our own grasping at transitory pleasures in a misguided attempt to escape mental and physical pain.

The Buddha identified four characteristics of suffering. The first of these characteristics is the suffering of impermanence. Within the realm of material existence there is nothing that does not change or pass away in time. Even empty space is continually altered by the changing nature of the things that occupy space. In spite of this obvious truth, human beings tend to grasp at impermanent things and conditions. Our grasping extends to feelings and concepts as well. Yet, try as we might, our grasping only ends in frustration and disappointment. We feel frustration when we fail to attain the desired object or condition. However, we also feel disappointment when we manage to obtain our desired object or condition. The excitement of possessing the desired object or condition soon fades. In the wake of this emotional fading we are left wanting more. It is this built-in tendency toward disaffection that the Buddha identified as dukkha.

The next form of suffering is base suffering or ordinary pain. Base suffering is programmed into animals by their own DNA. It is responsible for our need to constantly seek out new feeding and breeding grounds. Without base suffering an animal would lack the intrinsic motivation necessary for survival. Base suffering is so ingrained that it is easily overlooked as one of the underlying sources of distress. Nonetheless, it is also a powerful instinctual force that fuels our avariciousness.

Next on the list of the characteristics of suffering is what is understood in Buddhism as emptiness. The suffering of emptiness refers to the fact that all seemingly solid objects are made of energy and space. It is appealing to imagine that our new car has a kind of identity of its own. We imbue our shiny new vehicle with a soul that is also a badge of personal status and self-worth. But over time our excitement fades. Now we must cast about for some new possession onto which we can project our self-identity. We find ourselves, again and again, grasping for something 'real' in this world. Perhaps a lasting relationship will do the trick? Maybe we join a political cause or religious group with which we can identify? But nothing seems to satisfy our thirst. In our grasping we are attempting to, metaphorically speaking, catch the wind. And like the wind, the objects we cling to are just as devoid of an intrinsic self-nature. There is no car within the car to be found. There is only a collection of parts that interact to create the empty phenomenon that we label a 'car'. The same idea applies when we project a negative quality onto a given object. Suppose we were to trip over a tennis shoe that we failed to put back on the shoe rack after our morning run? Our instant reaction might be to think "Stupid shoe! What are you trying to do, kill me?" Now we are angry and resentful at a mindless tennis shoe! As silly as this sounds, it is an all too common reaction in life. We tend to act out of the misperception that objects have an intrinsic self-nature. This mistaken view often leads to lashing out at the 'bad' objects in our environment. We might hurl the offending tennis shoe across the room which results in a broken vase. In the end, of course, we are only hurting ourselves.

Understanding the emptiness of phenomena, we come to the fourth characteristic of suffering. This is the suffering of selflessness.

Just as there is no car within the car, neither is there a self-identity to be found within the mind or body. Upon close examination we fail to pin down a distinct self-entity that is supposedly operating behind the activities of the mind. If the 'self' is located somewhere in the brain, then where? Is the 'self' located in the front or back of the brain? Perhaps we can narrow the 'self' down to the higher brain functions? But which part of the higher brain? Using this approach we end up dividing and quartering only to divide and quarter again and again. And still the 'self' eludes us. Yet, of all of our attachments, primarily it is our grasping at the notion of a unique and irreducible 'self' that drives the engine of suffering. We project our self-identity into the past and then experience feelings of depression and regret. Conversely, we may project the 'self' into an imagined future and thereby generate feelings of anxiety or worry. In either case we miss the reality of the moment. But it is only in-the-moment – the here-and-now – that we have the power to do something about suffering.

As an exercise in non-attachment and experiential acceptance, I sometimes lead a client in what I call the ice cube exercise. The ice cube exercise is widely used in cases where the client turns to self-harm in order to garner a temporary release from emotional pain. People sometimes cut on themselves for the endorphin release. The pain prompts the body to respond with a release of natural pain killing neurotransmitters. There is often an element of masochism involved as well. The ice cube exercise provides the client with a safe way to generate the release of endorphins without resorting to mutilation. In Auto Process Therapy the element of mindful acceptance is introduced. The client is taught to experience the sensations of pain as waves that arise, abide, and then melt once again into the ocean of pure awareness. Pain is seen as being an empty and impermanent form of energy. In this way the client can begin to separate the experience of suffering from the pain signal. Suffering is grasping at pleasant sensations or, alternately, clinging to *not* experiencing unpleasant feelings. Taking the ice cube exercise one step further, the client can be led to experience grasping as another kind of mental wave. Since grasping leads to suffering, the extinction of suffering can be learned using the ice cube approach to increase one's capacity for acceptance and non-attachment, i.e., letting go.

Suffering can only exist in the past or the future. If we are truly mindful and accepting of our moment-to-moment experience it is impossible to suffer. We may feel pain; but, as stated before, pain is not the same as suffering. Looking with deep insight into our immediate experience we find nothing to cling to. Furthermore, there is no self who is grasping in the first place. Since there is nothing to cling to, there is no need to grasp. If there is no grasping, then there is no suffering born of grasping. This being said, the flow of mental images, feelings, and sensations passes so quickly it is hard to track. The cultivation of such a highly developed ability to see into the selfless reality of the moment comes only with training, consistent practice, methodical skill-building, and the cultivation of compassion for one's self.

Another way to think of grasping is that it is a form of resistance. Suffering comes into being as a result of our attempts to resist the raw, sensory data of pain. We also suffer by resisting the loss of pleasure. Resistance is a kind of mental tensing against a painful sensation or emotion. Quite often we tense against our thoughts and feelings in anticipation of an unpleasant experience. When we imagine undertaking an unpleasant task such as having a root canal we tense against the thought. On the other hand, when we consider attaining a desired goal such as going on a long anticipated trip to Hawaii we generate another kind of mental tensing. This tensing takes the form of craving. In either case we are adding an additional level of unpleasant feelings to our immediate experience. The sensation of cold is not as bad as when we tense against the cold. Only by relaxing into the cold do we begin to reduce our suffering. Opening to the painful experience is what is meant by acceptance. However, when we combine resistance with grasping and ignorance we generate the trifecta of suffering.

Central to maintaining the trifecta of suffering is the workings of the ego. The ego is not a self. Rather, the ego is an automated function within the mind. The role of the ego is to maintain a separate, autonomous sense of self. By doing so the ego can better ensure the basic survival needs of the human organism. Its core activity is to make order out of the unrefined sensory data that is transmitted via the five senses to the mind. The ego does this by taking control of what the mind is made aware of and how the mind interprets the raw information. At the end of the day it is the primary task of the ego to provide us with a sense of control over our reality. Problems occur when the ego function runs away from us by over-controlling all aspects of our lives. The ego operates on all levels of our consciousness and is extremely good at erecting defenses that are designed to maintain the illusion of separation. However, in doing so the ego often magnifies our suffering.

One of the ways that the ego controls the day to day operations of the mind is by creating mental objects. Mental objects are concepts that symbolize various aspects of our reality. A chair-object stands in for all objects in the category of chair. This ability of the mind is learned in early childhood and serves as a shorthand way for us to get our bearing. We also generate objects to stand in for other people. Objects of this nature are imbued with our own personality projections and often include cast-off parts of ourselves. The cast-off parts are made up of aspects of our personality that we try to disown. The danger is that we can use actual people as blank screens upon which we project negative parts of our own personalities. If taken to the extreme we might come to hate someone, not for who they really are or what they have done, but for what they have come to represent about ourselves. The beneficial function of mental objects is that they can serve as targets for the basic energy of the mind. When used in this way the mental object can ground otherwise harmful emotions such as rage, lust, or fear. Learning to recognize the way we use our mental objects can result in using our mental objects more effectively. For instance, we can generate a wholesome mental object and then radiate the associated positive feelings throughout our nervous system. The end result of this practice can produce many therapeutic benefits such as reduced hypertension, lower blood pressure, and a reduction in chronic pain.

With regard to the issue of resistance and craving, the common denominator that unites these energies is *tanha* or attachment. The impulses toward or against something passes very quickly. However, when we attach to the impulse we create craving or aversion. If we continue to feed our attachment we can easily slip into feelings of greed or hatred. All attachment is rooted in a fear of letting go. If I surrender my grasp on this or that I will be diminished in some way. I may experience pain and even death. I must hang on! But if the self that we are trying to defend does not actually exist then our attachments are already in vain. In order to maintain a stable sense of self the ego comes into play. One of the ways that the ego sustains the illusion of separation is by drawing on unconscious false beliefs or, as they are referred to in Buddhism, fetters.

The fetters are specific attachments that combine to keep us tied to false beliefs. If we think of a single string we have no problem breaking the hold that the string has on us. But when multiple strings are woven together we find ourselves bound by a rope of attachments. The fetters number ten in all and work to maintain a false representation of reality. The end result is to create five basic harmful states of mind called hindrances. They are hindrances because they limit our ability to be clear-minded and at ease. The five hindrances are: the mind of ill will or anger, the mind of worry and restlessness, the mind of sensual desire, the mind of torpor or laxness, and the mind of doubt.

The main thing to consider is that there is a reason for suffering and that pain is different from suffering. Suffering does not simply fall on us from on high. Rather, it is rooted in attachment born of our fundamental mistaken understanding of our self-nature and of reality. We attach to the notion of a separate self-identity and unconsciously project our self onto everything and everyone around us. But by doing so we are denying the fact of impermanence, selflessness, and emptiness of phenomena. Furthermore, we fail to understand that our very DNA is programmed for disaffection. No sooner do we attain the desired object or circumstances then we become restless and seek out new acquisitions. It is for this reason that APT first attempts to shine the light of awareness on the nature of suffering. Without having an understanding of the cause and effect nature of suffering we may come to despair of ever finding solutions to life's many challenges.

The Clinical Perspective

Beyond the root premise of no actual intrinsic (Object-Self) to be found, the bulk of Buddhist theory is concerned with (1) the four characteristics of suffering as delineated in the First Noble Truth, and (2) the conditions that give rise to the psychological state of suffering or dukkha, and, ultimately, the countermeasures to these conditions. For the purposes of the extinction of suffering, the Buddha singled out three interacting dynamics that Western psychotherapists would label as: addiction or greed "*lobha*", resistance or hatred "*dosa*", and ignorance or denial "*moha*", as being the necessary precursors to suffering. (Noss, 1999, p 176) Taken together, these three elements form the Buddhist cognitive-behavioral triad of suffering. (Appendix, Fig. 1) Generally speaking, the three countermeasures needed to extinguish suffering are: discernment or "*prajna*", effective moral and ethical action "*sila*", and the cultivation of direct insight into one's own self-nature "*samadhi*". (Bhikkhu Bodhi, 2005) Concerning the four characteristics of suffering, they are understood to be: the suffering of impermanence, base or ordinary suffering, the suffering of emptiness, and the suffering of selflessness. Therapeutically, the countermeasures to the causes of suffering are non-attachment in response to addiction, unconditional acceptance coupled with constructive action in response to resistance, and the development of insight and discrimination in the face of denial. The four characteristics of suffering describe the general symptoms that point to the diagnosis of the problem.

To better grasp the relationship between the conditions that give rise to suffering it is important to gain a better understanding of the nature and function of the ego. According to Buddhist theory the ego is not viewed as a subjective self but rather as a function of the mind. "The self-concept or ego is nothing more than a set of reactions and

47

mental images that are artificially pasted into the flowing process of pure awareness". (Gunaratana, 2011, p 24) This artificial pasting is accomplished, in the main, through the over-generalizing function of memory. One moment of self is linked to another at the level of synaptic connections in the brain to form a network of self-moments. The nature of these synaptic linkages is nothing other than memories formed since early childhood. The end result is that we are tricked into believing that we has some kind of unshakable permanency because we remember past, associated self-moments. Therefore, a primary task of the ego is to link individual self-moments together.

The ego serves to regulate and balance the various energies of the psyche, i.e., the Id, superego, cognitions, feelings, sensations, etc. "To Freud, the ego was the pragmatic executor. It was the agency needed to strike a workaday balance between the two [superego and Id]". (Austin, 2001, p. 35) The end result of the ego's balancing act between superego and Id is to generate a visceral feeling, as well as the idea of a self or the "I-Me-Mine" complex. "These three components interlock in a tight complex, each complementing the other". (Austin, 2001, p 44) In Auto Process Therapy, the ego function is seen as creating a variety of personality projections or internal "objects" that human beings begin to construct as small children in order to make sense of their environments. "One of the most important developments in the sensorimotor stage is the acquisition of the object concept". (Galotti, 1999, p 475) APT posits that these internal objects then interact as a means of channeling the unconscious psychic energies of aggression, desire, and anxiety (Appendix, Fig 4). If you have ever wondered why you spend a large part of each day carrying on internal discussions with imaginary people (self-objects) in your mind. . . this is one of the principle reasons.

As a regulating and balancing function the ego has a lot on its plate. Consequently, it behooves us to be grateful to the ego function for doing such an amazing job as our internal, psychological office manager. It is not uncommon for people to view the ego as some kind of bad guy. But nothing could be farther from the truth. It is only when the ego function is misunderstood that the ego can become a problem.

A closer examination of the ego function reveals that there is no *one* in the ego. Nor can we say that the ego is self-aware. Rather, the ego is only a blind, automatic mechanism in the mind that is devoid of life and self. In spite of the convincing otherness of our personality projections, they too are devoid of a self-nature. Objects Relations theorists focus on a particular function of the ego as it impacts how we relate to the people around us. "We relate to others on the basis of expectations formed by early experience. The residue of these early relationships leaves internal objects – mental images of self and other built up from experience and expectation". (M. Nichols, R. Schwartz, 2004, p. 230) These internal objects/personality projections act in an almost autonomous manner. In this sense they are like sub-personalities with little egos of their own. It is their seeming realness that compels us to spend so much energy interacting with these internal personality projections. And as the term personality *projection* implies, we also cast these internal self-objects onto the people and things around us. For this reason, it is imperative that we come to understand the true nature of our personality projections. If not, we risk going through life interacting with internal phantoms that have little to do with actual people. So convincing is our ability to project personality objects that we may fail to recognize how much we project feelings such as anger onto the people, things, and situations we encounter every day. It is as if the people in our environment serve as a blank screen upon which we cast our internal projections, for better or worse. Yet we can learn to stand back psychologically, in a manner of speaking; and in so doing, we can begin the process of forgiving ourselves for our natural shortcomings as human beings. It is by forgiving ourselves that we can heal our self-sabotaging behaviors, along with our relationships.

Another reason that we generate and interact with personality projections is to avoid the disquieting feeling of isolation. Human beings are social animals that depend upon each other for survival. The twin impulses to connect with other people and the drive towards self-preservation, compel us to avoid social isolation while seeking social support. In the absence of actual social contact we will invent people in our minds to interact with us. At times these pseudo social interactions serve as a useful form of cognitive rehearsal. But for the most part they take us away from fully experiencing the present moment.

From a therapeutic standpoint the skillful use of internal mental objects to transform emotions – from toxic to healthy ones – is both time honored and proven to be effective. From Western Object Relations Theory, to shamanistic vision quests and a variety of

Eastern meditation practices throughout the ages, the use of internal objects is a central element of healing and empowerment. Buddhist dharma teacher, Thich Nhat Hanh, points out that consciousness must be conscious of something, a mental object for instance, in order to exist at all. The way that the subject – in this example, ourselves – understands the object or that which we perceive, determines the corresponding emotional state we experience. With this idea in mind, the patient can be taught to become mindful of the objects he or she is generating at any given moment. Along with mindfulness of internal objects, the patient can also become cognizant of the feeling states associated with the objects. From this point the patient can alter his or her feeling state by either consciously generating a positive object or letting of the negative object. Having done so, the patient can learn to defuse the energy of the object by using breath work and imagination.

With regard to addiction and resistance (grasping and aversion), the ego is the master of attaching to things it finds self-reinforcing and resisting that which it finds threaten. The experience of pleasure is not, in itself, a harmful thing. However, the need to hold on to the experience of pleasure at all costs is at the very heart of addiction. The middle way school of Buddhism holds that both the self and phenomena are impermanent and utterly lacking in a fixed or static Object-Self nature (First Noble Truth). Therefore, any attempt to cling to the object of desire is doomed to fail. Such failure leads to disappointment and suffering. At this point, it is not uncommon for the ego to compel the self or "Sovereign I" to redouble its efforts to regain the perceived source of pleasure (Austin, 2001, p. 44). On the other hand, the ego may drive the self to seek out new and singular forms of pleasure. In either case, the cycle of addiction is activated. As for resistance, the ego can enlist a host of strategies in the form of defense mechanisms. Defense mechanisms are unconscious maneuvers on the part of the ego function designed to protect the mind from being unbalanced. Too much anxiety or aggression can topple the mind. For this reason the ego strives to always regulate intense feelings of anxiety and aggression. It is to this end that unconscious defense mechanisms are utilized. However, because defense mechanisms *are* unconscious they are also outside of our control. Normally this is not an issue except when defense mechanisms begin to work against us. At such a point it becomes necessary to bring the unconscious defense mechanisms into mindful awareness and either modify them or discard them altogether. Once having done so we can then replace the unconscious defense mechanisms with conscious, adaptive coping behaviors. As for resistance, in Buddhist psychology resistance is met with an accurate evaluation and unconditional acceptance of one's self and circumstances. Another manifestation of resistance is the pushing away of painful emotions and sensations. It is natural for an organism to protect itself by pulling away from painful stimuli. However, there are times when such stimuli cannot, or should not, be shut out. At such cases it is extremely dangerous to ignore the body's attempts to alert us to sickness or injury. As an alternative to ignoring the pain signal, in APT the client is taught to embrace painful stimuli with mindful acceptance. By utilizing the skill of unconditional acceptance it is possible to separate the pain signal from the state of suffering. In this way we can begin to replace suffering with equanimity. Marsha Linehan, the creator of dialectical behavioral therapy, framed the relationship between pain and suffering as a simple equation:

Pain (P) + Resistance (R) = Suffering (S). (P + R = S)

Therefore, **Pain (P) + Unconditional Acceptance (UA) = Equanimity (E)** even in the presence of physical or psychological pain. **(P+UA=E)**

The pain feedback signal may still be active; but due to unconditional acceptance the mind can remain in a state of psychological balance.

Returning briefly to the subject of how the ego function uses internal objects to regulate and balance the mind, it is important to note that the projected object serves as a target for anxiety, aggression, and desire. The object is generated from unconscious material that is almost always drawn from the experience of early caregivers. Objects can also be a representation of the child schema. Having created an object to serve as a target, the ego then projects the energies of aggression, anxiety, and desire at the externalized target. The target-object serves as one end of a pole that helps to ground powerful feelings of anxiety, aggression, or desire. At this point the object becomes active and sends the energy back to the unconscious mind thus creating a feedback loop (Appendix, Fig 4). The end result is to contain, and ultimately to dissipate, psychic energy and thus prevent the ego from being overwhelmed by emotion. An example might be that of mentally telling off one's employer. The act of conjuring up a mental object of our employer and then shouting at him serves to channel aggression that might otherwise be vented in harmful ways. By imagining shouting at our boss instead of actually doing so we are more likely to ensure that we retain our employment! On the other hand, when feelings of aggression, fear, or sadness are repressed entirely out of our conscious awareness they often surface as various forms of pathology. In extreme instances intense, unintegrated feelings of anxiety, aggression, and desire can topple the mind, as in the case of the psychotic patient. Once again, in APT, the ego function is seen as fulfilling a vital role in the regulation and balance of the mind. It is only when the function of the ego is not understood (unconsciousness) that it can fall back on maladaptive coping strategies. Such maladaptive coping strategies include alcohol and drug abuse, sexual misconduct, and all manner of reckless behavior. Becoming mindful of the role of internal objects affords us powerful methods for redirecting and integrating emotional energy.

With regard to the specific nature of the thought distortions that arise out of our unconscious false beliefs or schemas, Buddhism has identified ten "fetters" that must be removed in the path to full enlightenment (Gunaratana, 2001, p. 151). The ten fetters consist of attachments to a specific false belief and are divided into three groups corresponding to three distinct levels of psychological imbalance. The first three fetters consist of: belief in a permanent and independent self (Object-Self), doubt in the Noble Eightfold Path or treatment, and the belief in the efficacy of ritualized magical thinking or religious practices (superstition).

The next level of imbalance corresponds more to the subconscious mind. The fetters at this level are the unconscious attachment to the idea that life will be better if a desired materialistic goal can be attained. For instance, the client may fantasize about winning a lottery and never having to work again. Another example of the fetter of materialistic attainment is that one can find lasting happiness by finding the perfect job or partner. The other fetter associated with this level of imbalance is the desire to escape into a formless state such as going to the Christian Heaven or being born in the Buddhist Pure Land. In either case the client is investing in the attachment to an ideal state of existence that can never come to be. The more the client invests in these romantic scenarios the more dissatisfied they become with their current reality. Since these attachments are never brought into awareness they tend to churn away in the background of the client's consciousness. By contrast, with the first three fetters the client may be fully aware of their beliefs, however without understanding that such beliefs are distorted at best. It is at this level that we also encounter the fetters of resistance or ill will and addiction or sensual desire.

The remaining fetters are concerned with spiritual pride (narcissism), spiritual restlessness (existential anxiety), and ignorance of the process nature of the self and phenomenon in general (delusion). These fetters are deeply embedded in the unconscious and are the last to be addressed in therapy. In terms of stages of APT, these levels of imbalance articulate clearly defined treatment goals with regard to the phases of therapy. Of course, as therapists, we must also keep in mind the individual goals the patient has outlined for coming to therapy as well.

To summarize, the psychological state of suffering can be understood as being the result of the ego's efforts to avoid the experience of pain (resistance), acquire and possess unhealthy objects of desire (addiction), and remain unaware of the process nature of existence (denial). The underlying reason for the ego's mistaken attempts at pain avoidance and obsessive pleasure seeking is found in unconscious habits rooted in delusion. The chief delusion is the belief in the existence of an unchanging, eternal, and intrinsic self or Object-Self. Furthermore, suffering is understood as being a temporary psychological state of dissatisfaction that is distinct from pain. Pain is defined as being either physical or psychological in nature and as being a necessary form of feedback. As part of a feedback system pain alerts us to when we are out of balance. APT posits that suffering can be extinguished one moment at a time through a combined process of insight building and skill building. Insight building aims to gain understanding of unconscious blocks and to restructure the self-schema. The skill building aspect of APT serves to promote both emotional resilience and identity stability during the challenging process of cognitive restructuring. APT makes use of four behavioral skill sets that are divided into: insight skills (*samadhi*), ethical behavior skills (*karma*), discernment skills (*prajna*), and emotional regulation skills (*bodhicitta*).

Lastly, with regard to pathological states of mind, Buddhism identifies five basic types or hindrances that are delineated as: greed, ill-will, dullness (torpor), worry and restlessness, and doubt (Gunaratana, 2001). From the point of view of APT these pathological mind states can be understood as addiction (greed), resistance (ill-will), denial (dullness), anxiety (worry and restlessness), and depression (doubt). These five pathological states of mind arise when one or more of the underlying unconscious fetters are activated. In terms of cognitive behavioral theory the fetters can be considered maladaptive, unconscious beliefs. Therefore, the insight building aspect of APT includes raising the fetters into the light of conscious awareness. When elevated to the level of awareness they can be countered with advanced coping behaviors. By integrating insight building with skill building in both an individual and group setting, the APT therapist seeks to help the patient to arrive at and sustain a Process-Self perspective. This perspective is flexible enough to allow for growth and change and yet stable enough to adapt to the inevitable crises, stressors, and challenges of life.

Chapter Four
The Path of Liberation

"Suffering do I teach; and the way out of suffering" — Buddha

The Layperson's Perspective

Imagine for a moment that you are a fully awakened being. In your ongoing state of enlightenment you experience all of your thoughts, feelings, perceptions, and sensations as an unending stream of energy. You are at peace and fully engaged in a moment-to-moment process of living, expressing, and radiating selfless core awareness. You are like a brilliant light that gives forth rays of infinite intelligence and boundless compassion. You are a Buddha.

To other people you seem perfectly ordinary as you stand in line at the movie theater or browse the aisles of a bookstore. There is nothing to distinguish you from any other person on earth other than your calm smile or kind eyes. Perhaps if we were to take a closer look we would see that your movements seem more relaxed and integrated than other people. You give off an air of being alert and aware yet not hypervigilant. On the inside you exist in a state of non-attached acceptance and equanimity. If a moment of anger, fear, or sadness arises it quickly passes like a wave melting back into the ocean. Your internal, discursive thinking patterns are almost non-existent. Your mind is open and free of mental clutter like a vast and luminous sky. Your sense of self is little more than a reflection that plays on the surface of a sea of pure awareness. Yours is an all-inclusive peace that allows for the full range of human experience without being caught up in any of it. No, you are not superhuman – rather, you are fully human.

In theory any of us can become such an awakened being. All that stands in our way are deeply entrenched, destructive patterns of thinking, feeling, and behaving. These patterns are habitual mental scripts that capture our attention and distract us from our core awareness. They operate largely in the background of consciousness and are rooted in a profound misunderstanding of reality. There are many such destructive scripts and in every instance they are fueled by attachment and grasping. Attachment gives rise to craving and aversion which then activates even more scripts. In this way the momentum of suffering continues from birth to rebirth, one moment to the next. When we are caught up in a destructive script we might say to ourselves, "I deserve to be treated with more respect!" The next step in this sequence is to tense up internally, by grasping at a mental picture of ourselves as a victorious hero fighting off attackers. We imagine telling off the person who we think is mistreating us. Now we act out in some minor but unhealthy way such as throwing a book across the room or pouring ourselves a drink. We begin to ruminate about all the times in our lives when other people mistreated us, and we stew in our juices of resentment. But what if, through a process of uncovering and letting go of our destructive mental scripts, we can begin to achieve a shift in perspective? Perhaps we can formulate and integrate new mental scripts that foster feelings of peace and friendship. In this process of integration we might begin by becoming mindful of our habitual patterns of thinking and feeling. We discover that each of our patterns has a feeling tone that either draws us towards, or propels us away, from a given set of people and circumstances. In other cases our scripts have a dull or neutral feeling tone. If a homeless person crosses our path on the way to work our judgement script becomes activated. We might then run through a sequence of thoughts resulting in a feeling of apathy. Our script ends, as it always does, with the thought, "There is nothing I can do." We might run an anger script that begins with the thought, "Why don't these people just get it together?" And, at the end of a series of verbal statements and mental images, we conclude, "You can't fix the world!" Our feeling tone is angry and the mind of ill-will arises to hinder our ability to be non-attached, present, and kind.

Auto Process Therapy assumes that we are all capable, in various degrees, to become more aware of our destructive mental habits and of changing them. APT also concedes that the effort of uncovering our hidden mental scripts is both challenging and unrealistic without the help of a trained teacher or therapist. Whereas the goal of Buddhism is the final extinction of suffering and the awakening to ultimate reality, APT has as its goals the moment-to-moment extinction of suffering and the empowerment to greater peace. Yet this is not to say that the goal of supreme enlightenment is too lofty to pursue. On the contrary, the goal of enlightenment is fully supported by the APT therapist if that is what the client is interested in. But along the way to ultimate enlightenment the client would be well served to learn and master the behavioral skill-building strategies that are an integral aspect of APT.

Along with mastering the skill-building strategies, the client will also benefit from the insight building aspects of APT that form the basis of individual therapy. Through insight building, a client can learn to recognize and activate their latent behavioral potentials or *bindus*/seeds of enlightenment. In this manner they may come to understand and experience their process nature of free flowing ease and grace. Ultimately, they may come to realize that the answers they were seeking outside of themselves lay within.

In the coming chapters we will explore the methods utilized in APT for helping a client to uncover, restructure, and remove unwholesome patterns of thinking, feeling, and behaving. We will also explore the therapeutic maneuvers used in APT to help a client to intuitively recognize and express their deeper nature or core awareness. It is through this back and forth learning method that a client can realize and actualize a profound shift in their worldview from the Object-Self to the Process-Self perspective.

The Clinical Perspective

In my work as a therapist I have discovered that the twin objectives "to be happy" and "to be free from suffering" are rarely the primary reasons the client seeks out counseling. More often than not, the client's goal is to gain a greater feeling of control in some area of their life. It is here that we must be careful not to equate self-interest with the feeling of happiness, let alone inner peace. Self-interest can take many forms and result in a variety of emotional outcomes. With regard to the ego function, the emotional outcome is always linked to a feeling of personal power. This is to say that on an ego function level self-interest plays out as achieving a feeling of control. However, personal power – as a feeling state – is not the same as happiness. Nor can we say that the feeling of control is equal to the absence of suffering. The ego is a powerful mental apparatus that does not care about happiness or suffering; rather, it is only interested in survival. Therefore, the primary function of the ego is to keep us alive by attempting to control every aspect of our existence.

For the client to express a desire to be free from suffering and be happy represents a significant step towards giving up their symptoms. Having established the desire to overcome suffering and to be happy, it is then essential to take a closer look at the causes and conditions that give rise to suffering and happiness.

Simply put, suffering is due to our own delusional thinking born of ignorance. Because of delusion we are attached to, and desire, an object-self that does not actually exist. This attachment generates addiction to pleasure, resistance to that which is painful, and denial concerning our own underlying nature of selfless mutability. Addiction, resistance, and denial give rise to such toxic emotions as anger, fear, and desire. Therefore, seeing through to the process side of reality is the beginning of liberation from suffering. The selfless nature of reality is referred to in Buddhism as emptiness. "Selflessness or emptiness is reality, not a doctrinal belief created by the Buddha". (Tserling, 2009, p. 6) APT posits that liberation from the state of suffering depends on following a treatment program that replaces addiction with non-attachment, resistance with unconditional acceptance, and denial with insight into reality (Appendix, Fig. 2). In the Four Noble Truths and the Noble Eightfold Path – upon which the APT skill-building modules are predicated – the Buddha outlines such a path to liberation.

Buddhism argues that, because of the law of impermanence, life as we typically live it is a set-up for disappointment and frustration. Thus, the Buddha's First Noble Truth states that all of life is suffering or "*dukkha*" (Noss, 1999, p. 179). Therefore, the more we cling to that which is inherently impermanent, the more we will experience suffering or anguish. It is in accepting unconditionally the fact of impermanence that we begin to embrace the reality principle. Failure to do so will manifest in any number of symptoms born of addiction, resistance, and denial. In our assessment of the problem we can then conclude that the patient is in pain because they misunderstand and deny the facts of impermanence, emptiness, and selflessness. If a client clings to some fixed notion of how she or he *should* have been (past), *must* be (present), or *has* to be (future), they become mired in delusion and suffering. Now we can assign a diagnosis by identifying the specifics of the patient's addiction, resistance, and denial of the aforementioned facts of impermanence, process, and selflessness.

The remaining characteristics of the First Noble Truth of suffering are: base suffering, the suffering of emptiness, and the suffering of selflessness. "In the Mahayana tradition, each noble truth possesses four characteristics, making sixteen in all. Commentaries such as the Ornament of Clear Realization *(Abhisamayalamkara)* by Maitreya explain these characteristics as a meditation guide to be practiced during the path to enlightenment". (Tserling, 2005, p. 42) For our purposes as clinicians, it may be helpful to include these subtle aspects of suffering in formulating our diagnosis of the patient's stated complaint.

Base or gross suffering is what we normally think of as suffering. This is suffering arising from chronic pain and discomfort. It is predicated upon our DNA's programmed reaction to avoid pain. As such, it is a function of the body's instinct for self-preservation. The APT therapist might suggest the cultivation of unconditional acceptance as a starting point when addressing gross suffering. On a more subtle level, it is base suffering that is the cause of our innate dissatisfaction. Animals are programmed by genetic factors to be restless as a survival mechanism. It is this innate restlessness that drives an animal to seek out new hunting and breeding grounds. The human animal is no exception. Were it not for base suffering we might find it difficult to compete in life. Unfortunately, base suffering also plays a central role in addiction and craving.

The suffering of emptiness refers to the fact that all phenomena are empty of an eternal self-nature. Emptiness of phenomena is closely related to the suffering of impermanence but goes more deeply into the process nature of reality. Not only do we cling, out of delusion and ignorance, to that which is impermanent; but we also cling to empty effects as if they were solid and fixed in nature. The cultivation of the skill of accurate analysis might be a good starting point in helping the patient to reframe their views on Object-Self versus Process-Self.

Lastly we return to the nature of our own personal self-nature. It is here that we encounter the suffering of selflessness. The suffering of selflessness, like the suffering of impermanence and emptiness, is rooted in our misapprehension of our own identity as being fixed, eternal, and unchanging. It is this aspect of suffering that is most responsible for human suffering in general.

Taken together, the four characteristics of the truth of suffering present a formidable challenge to overcome. Yet, underlying these four aspects of suffering is the deep-seated belief in the existence of fixed, eternal, and unchanging objects. Chief among these objects is the Object-Self. It is for this reason that APT makes it the fundamental goal of therapy to achieve a profound shift in perception away from the Object-Self. In place of the Object-Self, the client is guided to realize a Process-Self perspective that is unhooked from the past or the future. It is this shift that eventually leads to an integration of the Object-Self and the Process-Self perspectives.

Having assessed the situation, the Second Noble Truth states that the origin of suffering is destructive, unconscious habits that are rooted in delusions. This is to say that suffering does not simply fall upon us from out of the blue. Rather, is inexorably rooted in causal factors. It is, therefore, the truth of cause and effect that speaks to the diagnosis we formulate to describe the nature of the patient's complaint. To this end, the therapist must help the client to identify the antecedents of the problem; and along with the antecedents to the problem behaviors, the reinforcing behaviors that serve to maintain the problem after the fact. It is in understanding the role of internal cause and effect that the patient begins to gain a greater sense of personal autonomy with respect to their symptoms.

With regard to the formulation of a diagnosis there are three general categories for mental illness: thought disorders, mood disorders, and personality/behavior disorders. Other disorders are categorized under childhood disorders, medically-related disorders, substance abuse disorders, and so on. But in one way or the other, all disorders can be linked back to maladaptive interactions between thoughts, feelings, and interactions of individuals and groups of people. "Family relationships, cognitions, emotions, and behavior are viewed as exerting mutual influence on one another". (Nichols and Schwartz, 2004) Therefore, many forms of mental illness can be traced back to underlying causal factors and conditions. Central to these causes and conditions are maladaptive interactions between people.

The Third Noble Truth states that the cessation of suffering is an obtainable possibility. What this means, for both clinicians and patients, is that there is always hope. By adopting a hopeful point of view we begin to reorient the patient towards a solution-focused perspective. It is at this point that we can begin to formulate, in collaboration with the patient, the long-term goals of therapy and a treatment plan. The Third Noble Truth, then, can be said to mark the desired outcome of therapy.

Finally we arrive at the Fourth Noble Truth that is also the Noble Eightfold Path. It is here that we guide the patient through the process of therapy that is guided by our assessment, diagnosis, behavioral interventions, and treatment planning.

Although Auto Process Therapy utilizes a solution-focused and skill-based approach, APT is not, strictly speaking, a skill-based form of therapy. It does, however, depend on teaching the patient a variety of behavioral coping skills that are divided between insight skills, behavior skills, discernment skills and emotional regulation skills. Each of these groups of skill sets is referred to as a module. Yet, even though separated into specific modules, they are to be learned and integrated in tandem rather than in a strict sequential manner. For this reason the Process-Self is at the center of all four modules like the center of a flower that is surrounded by the flower's petals. The decision to focus on any one of the four APT modules as a starting point depends upon the needs and goals of the patient.

An emphasis on cognitive behavioral skill-building is important to APT. This being stated, as a therapy APT more aptly falls under the umbrella of the process schools of psychotherapy. The very name, Auto Process Therapy, speaks to the focus on process as being central to this approach. Suffering is not a static thing in time and space but rather a conditional state of mind subject to change. Likewise, liberation from suffering is also to be considered within the framework of APT as a state of being that is subject to change. As to the final extinction of suffering after death (*parinirvana*), APT takes no position. It is enough to manage mental anguish on a moment-to-moment basis for the goals of Auto Process Therapy to be met.

The APT therapist begins with assessment, proceeds to diagnosis, treatment planning, and finally the implementation of the therapeutic progression. The central aim of therapy is the reorientation by the client from the Object-Self perspective – with its attachment to pleasure and resistance to pain – to the Process-Self perspective that is unhooked from addictive attachments, pathological resistance, and the depression from the past or anxiety about the future. Along with these goals that are inherent to APT, the patient and the therapist will work together to identify specific goals connected to the patient's life circumstances.

Part two of this book will focus on the stages of APT and the therapeutic maneuvers most commonly used by the APT therapist. APT is conceived to take a combined individual and group therapy approach. This is because of the emphasis APT places on behavioral skill-building and practical application. The feedback provided by other patients who are using APT in their lives is critical to the mastery of APT's four behavioral coping modules. Although APT draws on any number of psychotherapeutic perspectives, one cannot be said to practice APT divorced from its root premise of there being no separate self-entity. Lastly, APT is an ongoing form of therapy rather than a brief therapy. APT can and should be taken in prescribed amounts over time. The journey from Object-Self to Process-Self is a lifelong one. For this reason, APT should be viewed as part of lifelong integration of the Object- and Process-Self perspective.

APT Stages of Therapy: Recognition, Acceptance, Hope, and Treatment.

First Noble Truth (Suffering). Recognition.

The patient is prompted to investigate the nature of both their personal suffering and suffering in general. This is the stage of recognition of the problem.

The Second Noble Truth (Origin of Suffering). Acceptance.

The patient gains a greater sense of personal agency, i.e., internal locus of control, regarding suffering by understanding their role in creating and maintaining personal delusions, toxic emotions, and destructive cognitive-behavioral habits or scripts. This is the stage of acceptance of their role in the problem.

The Third Noble Truth (Liberation). Hope.

The patient gains a clear understanding of what mental health looks like for them and that mental health is a real possibility. The patient begins to form an internal working model based on accurate understanding, equanimity, compassion, kindness, and positive behavioral habits.

The Fourth Noble Truth (Path). Treatment.

The patient has integrated the APT behavioral coping skills and gained significant insight into the Process-Self. At this stage the patient has a command of the treatment method and can consistently apply the goals and means of treatment to everyday l

Part Two
Auto Process Therapy:
Therapeutic Maneuvers
And Stages of Therapy

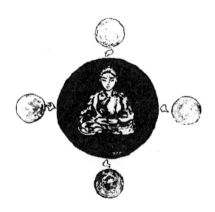

Chapter Five
Stages of Auto Process Therapy and APT Therapeutic Maneuvers

*"Failure is the key to success; each mistake
teaches us something new" –
Morihei Ueshiba O Sensei; The Art of Peace*

The Layperson's Perspective

It is not uncommon for people to seek a simple, magic bullet solution to life's most complex problems. "If I could only win the Lottery then my problems would go away." But if you were to come into a sudden windfall would you be prepared to handle the repercussions of instant wealth? You might very easily find yourself fending off an army of people trying to raise money for one good cause or another. Distant relatives might show up demanding that you share the wealth because, after all, you *are* family. You may need an accounting firm to find creative ways to shield your money from the Internal Revenue Service. You would certainly be forced to take extra security measures to protect yourself and your family from criminals. Friends may come to resent you for your good fortune. At the end of the day you may find that monetary wealth does not bring you inner peace, wisdom, or boundless love. In point of fact, Buddhism would argue that the pursuit of material wealth simply feeds our feelings of craving and attachment. In feeding these feelings we only magnify our suffering in life and obscure our light of inner peace and joy. Once again, our magic bullet solution lets us down or makes matters worse than before! It is at this point that many people will up the ante by throwing more of the same at the problem and expecting a different result. "If I can only make another million dollars I can relax, and my problems will disappear." But even another million dollars in the bank does not buy us the ability to let go of worry, anger, or sadness. For this we need something more subtle and profound. We need insight.

If we look with deep mindfulness and accurate understanding into our problems we begin to see that most of our suffering stems from how we react to external circumstances. It is not the blaring car horn that is the origin of our anger. Rather, it is the chain of habitual mental reactions that is the problem. If we were in a state of calm and mindful awareness the sound of the horn would pass through our mind like sunlight through a pane of glass. But because of a lifetime of habit we push away the experience of the moment while clinging to the idealized picture of how the moment *should* be. It is in clinging to our imagined, perfect worldview that resistance and suffering arises. But our worldview is hidden in our unconscious mind, leaving us wondering why such a minor incident can propel us into a state of anger? We begin to wonder if there is something fundamentally wrong with who we are inside. Yet, try as we might, we cannot seem to pin down a self that can be mended in the first place. All the while we are attaching to an idealized vision of life that we can never achieve. To add to our confusion, our idealized vision is largely unconscious and out of touch with reality. In the end we run the risk of becoming neurotic, depressed, and anxious to the point of impairment. It is at this point that many people seek out professional help.

The APT approach to counseling offers a combination of therapeutic maneuvers and cognitive behavioral skill-building. Therapeutic maneuvers differ from therapeutic techniques in that they are more adaptive to the client's particular life circumstances than a simple technique. Therapeutic maneuvers do not force the client into making behavioral changes. Instead, they offer guidance while putting the elements of choice and control back in the hands of the client. Quite often the difference between a therapeutic technique and a maneuver lies in the intent of the practitioner. The APT therapist assumes that the client is the ultimate authority with regard to their own growth and healing. This stance is founded upon the central premise of Buddhism that we are all sleeping Buddhas on a journey of awakening. Underlying the various layers of our consciousness is a ground of being, our Buddha Nature, that is selfless, wise, and filled with compassion. In APT the ground of being is called core awareness. From time to time we have an intuition of core awareness when we feel as if we are in touch with an intelligence greater than ourselves. But because of our fundamental misunderstanding of reality and years of destructive mental scripts, we are unable to maintain our tenuous link to core awareness. Even if our eyes open for a moment they quickly close again. If we know what to look for we can take something of our momentary awakening experience into our conscious mind. But most people will dismiss such moments as interesting but unimportant anomalies that have no real relevance. But to the APT therapist such moments are opportunities to delve deeper into the Process-Self perspective.

Along the way to gaining insight into core awareness, the client is taught various methods of managing and integrating challenging emotions. Afflictive emotions have the power to derail our attempts to be mindful and kind. The skills of emotional integration and refinement offer important methods for neutralizing and transforming harmful emotions. Emotional integration consists of engaging the emotion with mindful acceptance until it returns to the overall totality of the mind. In this way the emotion is like a wave in the ocean that arises, abides, and subsides back into a neutral state. If we fight against the wave, we only make more waves and exhaust ourselves in the process. This would be analogous to throwing a stone into the pond in an attempt to chase away the ripples. But by simply observing the emotional wave from a position of relaxed acceptance the wave is instantly changed. Emotional refinement takes this method one step further by extracting the wholesome aspect of the afflictive emotion and putting it to a constructive use. Using this method we can first allow the emotion to integrate into a more manageable state. Once the emotion/wave subsides we can notice and expand into the wholesome aspect of the emotion. For instance, within the emotion of fear we can extract the positive quality of awareness. Anger can be refined into a feeling of focused purpose or determination. Sadness can become compassion for others who may be enduring similar challenges to our own. Anxiety can be refined into excitement, and the feeling of restlessness – which is a common hindrance to sitting meditation – into energy. Much depends on our learning to see past our mental pictures to the deeper reality beyond. In APT this skill is called Direct Experiential Realization (of reality). An emotion can be reduced to a label that can be further categorized as a "good" feeling or a "bad" feeling. But if we look, with the eye of insight and wisdom, we might discover that our good and bad feelings are actually part of a complex pattern of energy. What we decide to do with this energy – for better or worse – is up to us.

The Clinical Perspective

Even before the assessment phase of therapy, the APT therapist must remain firmly rooted in APT's foundation premise of no distinct, intrinsic self. And along with this premise, the clinician must also remember that the APT therapist does not fall back on therapeutic techniques or other control strategies. Instead, the APT therapist utilizes therapeutic maneuvers to guide the client to discover their own inner strengths and resources. The rationale for this is that in APT the emphasis is on the process aspects of therapy rather than the content areas. A patient can fail in the execution of a therapeutic technique; however, if the patient is seen as being in an ongoing process of healing then every application of the therapeutic maneuver – even when performed incorrectly – becomes an opportunity for learning and growth. Therefore, APT is a process therapy that leads a patient through the stages of therapy in which every misstep is seen as a teachable moment.

Like other forms of therapy, APT begins with standard practices including referrals, rapport building, information gathering, management practices, and attending to crisis and other safety issues. Beyond these considerations the APT therapist must determine if APT is a suitable therapeutic modality for the patient. Not all patients are capable of, or interested in, letting go of the Object-Self perspective. Ethically, the therapist must assess if his or her therapeutic approach is a good fit for the patient. Having determined that the patient might benefit from APT, the next step would be to educate the patient about the theory and goals of Auto Process Therapy. It is here that the goals of the patient must dovetail into the overall goals inherent in APT.

Once the initial stage goals and objectives of therapy are met the APT therapist will guide the patient into the middle phase of therapy. At this point the therapist begins to introduce to the patient the concept of the therapeutic maneuver.

A *maneuver* differs from a *technique* in its intent. A therapeutic technique is a specific method of bringing the mind under some measure of control. The APT maneuver, by contrast, is a way to guide the natural processes of the mind. It is a strategy that is flexible enough to be tailored to the unique needs and particular life challenges of the client. In APT it is understood that the mind cannot be directly controlled. The reason for this is that much of what is held as true by the conscious self is influenced by irrational beliefs hidden in the unconscious mind. This is to say, what we experience as our everyday self is like the tip of the proverbial iceberg jutting out of the sea. Most of the iceberg remains beneath the dark waters of the unconscious. In a larger sense, APT posits that life cannot be placed under our direct control because there are simply too many variables to manage. Some might argue that we can bring a measure of our life under our power of choice and control. This may be a valid point if taken in the context of acting *as if* there is an actual self (Object-Self); nonetheless, the overarching goal of APT is to make the shift from Object-Self to Process-Self. From the perspective of the Process-Self there is no need to control reality, and there is no *one* to control reality in the first place. This being said, because we have egos and physical bodies that appear to move through linear time and space, we must live life with a foot in two worlds, as it were. Therefore, a middle stage goal of APT is for the patient to learn to negotiate the dialect between two given extremes. In the case of control versus helplessness, the therapeutic synthesis consists of *guiding* one's life in an ongoing process of change and growth.

Returning to the therapeutic maneuver, it is critical that the therapist emphasizes the differences between technique and maneuver. In APT, there are two basic psychological types of maneuver: the cognitive-behavioral maneuver and the "meta" cognitive-behavioral therapeutic maneuver. Cognitive-behavioral maneuvers are squarely aimed at how our actions, intentional thinking, and communication patterns impact feeling. The term meta-cognitive refers to positioning ourselves above (meta) the cognitions of the mind. "Meta-cognition consists of cognition about one's own cognition" (Galotti, 1999, p. 505).

Along with meta-cognition, the therapist will familiarize the patient with learning theory. The rationale is that, in learning about the processes involved in knowledge acquisition, the client can increase their problem solving ability. It is here, in the area of learning about learning itself, that the field of meta-cognition has made the most inroads. Generally speaking, meta-cognition has identified two phases of learning that can be thought of as engaging in a conscious, ongoing evaluation of one's content learning – along

71

with the ability to implement procedural learning. Content learning refers to breaking down the information into identifiable parts and answers the question, what? Procedural learning looks at the sequence of steps necessary in order to solve the problem. Procedural learning is concerned with acquiring new skills and answers the question, how? Having integrated the content and process knowledge, one then applies it to the task at hand. APT recognizes that these fundamental components of learning are embedded in the acquisition and mastery of any new skill. This being so, the APT therapist seeks to make the patient aware of this fact early on in the process of therapy. In this way the patient is better predisposed to integrate APT maneuvers and apply them to real life situations.

The termination phase of therapy looks much like most standard forms of therapy. There is a review of gains made throughout the therapeutic process. Any remaining referrals to appropriate collaterals, agencies, and support groups are made. An aftercare plan and, if necessary, a safety plan is designed with the patient's input. Long-term follow up sessions are scheduled, and feelings associated with the end of therapy are addressed.

In the next chapters I will describe therapeutic maneuvers specific to Auto Process Therapy. Central to APT are meta-cognitive distancing maneuvers and the learning of the four behavioral skill sets around which APT is focused. The meta-goal of making the psychological shift in perspective from Object-Self to Process-Self runs throughout all three phases of therapy.

Stages of Auto Process Therapy

1. Beginning stage:
- Assessment
- Problem identification and crisis management
- Determine if APT is a suitable therapeutic modality
- Initial referrals (medical, psychiatric, etc.)
- Treatment plan

2. Middle Stage:
- Group skill-building
- Therapeutic maneuvers
- Insight building

3. Termination Stage:
- Review of progress made during treatment
- Referrals
- Maintenance plan

APT Therapeutic Maneuvers

In the practice of Auto Process Therapy it is important to emphasize that there are no APT therapeutic techniques. Rather, APT relies on therapeutic maneuvers, skill building, and insight building to empower the patient in a process of healing and growth. As stated before, a technique is a control tactic and runs the risk of becoming a form of manipulation on the part of the therapist. The hidden assumption is that the therapist, by right of his or her knowledge, training, and education, ultimately knows what is best for the patient. Often in this scenario the patient is seen as being in resistance to change and therefore needs, for his or her own good, to be guided in the direction of health and growth. But in APT everything is laid out in the open for the patient to see. If there is ego resistance, then the therapist points this fact out to the patient as being a natural and healthy function of the ego. In the course of identifying and changing deeply ingrained behavioral habits the client will often encounter resistance on both the internal and external fronts. On the internal front resistance comes in the form of the extinction burst. On the external front the client will encounter resistance from the family or group system. Family or group resistance happens as the family system seeks to maintain homeostasis. It does not matter that the family homeostasis is working to maintain suffering and unhealthy roles. Any change increases pressure to the system, be it our own internal psychological system or that latent with the group itself. In the case of APT interventions and the therapeutic process, the therapist takes an egalitarian stance so as to better align with the patient in the tradition of the humanist therapist. This approach is not a condemnation of other more directive therapies; rather, it is one that assumes that people have a natural tendency towards growth and balance along with the inner resources to succeed. In Buddhism this perspective is referred to as Buddha Nature. In this sense Buddha Nature speaks to our latent potential towards balance, growth, and self-realization. "In a deeper and yet more ordinary dimension, all of us are Buddha" (Aitken, 1982, p. 67).

One of the most common – and often misunderstood – practices in Buddhism is that of counting, or in some way being mindful of one's breathing. For the beginner breath counting is a recommended approach in that it better anchors the mind in-the-moment and keeps the practitioner honest. The task of counting our breaths forces us to be cognizant of the degree of our state of mindfulness. In my own practice in Zen Buddhism I was instructed to count my breath in sets of ten. After a time I was then told to keep track of the sets of ten breaths. This went on for many years with me struggling in my efforts to keep track. It was not until many years later that I discovered that the goal was to let go of controlling the breath in my practice of zazen. Letting go of technique, in this case breath counting, then opened the way for a deeper and more natural experience for meditation and greater personal insight.

When instructing a new client in breath counting it is helpful to frame the maneuver as being the initiation into a process rather than being a mental task. There is no value in counting one's breaths for the sake of performing a mental task. In fact, if breath counting is viewed as a control tactic it runs the danger of becoming an obsession in the mind of the client. In APT, breath counting is taught as being a useful and enjoyable exercise in being mindful. Ideally, the counting goes on in the background and serves to help the client to gain a degree of psychological distance from upsetting feelings and counterproductive thinking. At the same time, the practice of breath counting helps the client to gain the meta-cognitive overview with regard to their own mind.

The meta-cognitive overview is one in which the patient can become aware of the various functions and operations of the mind from a safe distance, psychologically speaking. From this perspective the patient can both participate in, and distance himself from, the ego function and cognitions of the mind. The meta-cognitive overview is the natural stance of the APT therapist and, to some extent, it is taught to the patient. But it is not, generally speaking, a goal of most forms of traditional therapy. APT, as opposed to traditional therapies, considers teaching the meta-overview as critical to the patient's ongoing mental health. Lacking the ability to get above the mind the patient is likely to be caught up in repetitive, maladaptive mental habits and behaviors (karma). APT posits that the more the patient learns to step back and objectively observe and label the operations of the mind, the more the patient can understand and to manage the overall functions of the mind.

Even before the maneuver of breath counting is introduced it is best to coach the patient in the concept of non-judgmentally observing their immediate experience. The skill of non-judgmental observation is a key element of mindfulness training. "Mindfulness is broken down into two major components by Linehan: the 'what skills' of observing, describing, and participating, and the 'how skills' of taking a non-judgmental stance, focusing on one thing in-the-moment and using skillful means" (Marra, 2005, p. 188). Because some patients will be connecting with their current experience threatening – as in the case of posttraumatic stress disordered clients – it is always best to teach mindfulness exercises in the safety of the therapeutic milieu. In this way mindfulness training can serve as a powerful method to enrich a patient's ongoing experience of life. Equally, if not more important, the skillful application of mindfulness can serve to better inoculate patients against distressful emotions by decreasing maladaptive escape and avoidance defenses. "Escape and avoidance behaviors take a lot of psychological energy and in fact avoidance and escape may actually define the process of agony itself" (Marra, 2005, p. 185). To this end, instructing the patient to focus on the feeling of their feet pressing against the ground or on their breathing is recommended should the patient become agitated or panic. Once the patient becomes confident with sitting in the experience of their current circumstances, it is then safe to teach breath counting along with other common mindfulness behaviors.

Breath counting is a standard practice in many forms of meditation and is often used in the Zen Buddhist practice of zazen. Za means to sit and Zen means to be awake. Therefore, zazen means to sit in a completely awake state of mind. "Sitting in clear-minded, open-eyed zazen, one develops the capacity to let go, and this gradually flows on into all other activities of one's daily life practice" (Austin, 2001, p. 14). As simple as this sounds, sitting in this way for even as brief a period of time as twenty minutes can be extremely challenging. In a Japanese zendo (place of training) very little actual instruction is given. Traditionally the teacher gives the students a set of instructions and only provides advice in formal, one-on-one sessions. Little in the way of group discussion is allowed, and other than during formal instruction with a teacher, students are left to discover the method of zazen on their own. For purposes of APT, the goal is to lead the patient through every stage of therapy until he or she has mastered the behavioral skills and maneuvers. APT is a form of therapy and not a religion or spiritual practice. Unlike the teacher of Zen Buddhist Meditation, the APT therapist does not seek to be seen as a guru or spiritual advisor. As stated before, from the APT standpoint, breath counting is taught as a way to create psychological distance from painful emotional and physical sensations. Likewise, it is also utilized as a powerful means of generating a state of non-attachment to aversive stimuli. "But suppose, with training, we become non-attached to distractions and learn to dampen these wild, emotional swings on either side of equanimity. Then we can enter that serene awareness, which is the soil for positive, spontaneous personal growth, often called spiritual growth." (Austin, 2001, p. 13)

With regard to the state of non-attachment versus detachment, in the non-attached state the patient is engaged with his or her current experience without clinging to any particular aspect of it. The state of non-attachment is referred to as *vairaigya* in Buddhism. In the state of detachment, by contrast, the patient is separated psychologically from the experience of the moment. Neither state is, in itself, better than the other; but rather one state can be more adaptive than the other depending on one's motives. In APT, detachment can be a precursor to non-attachment if taught in the right context. However, detachment can also be utilized as a means to dissociate from threatening feelings and sensations. It is at such times that it degenerates into a maladaptive defense mechanism. The APT therapist uses the psychological states of detachment and non-attachment in the service of teaching the patient meta-cognitive coping behaviors.

The means of learning and practicing non-attachment are varied but the essential thing is to stress the utility of such methods to the patient. Often, when in the grip of powerful emotions, a patient is more prone to act out in destructive ways. But by learning and employing a few meta-cognitive distancing maneuvers, the patient can regain a sense of choice and autonomy over their feelings. To this end, mindful breath counting or simply observing one's breathing can be of great value. More will be said on the skill of non-attachment in chapter seven, The Reprocessing Maneuver. For the purposes of learning a useful and simple method for creating psychological balance, the ancient practice of observing one's breath cannot be overstated.

Finally, APT utilizes six essential emotional management methods: cognitive reframing, non-attachment to emotions and feelings, accelerated emotional integration (AEI), emotional refinement, redirection/channeling (sublimation) of emotions, and paradoxical intentionality (PI). Much of the *bodhicitta* or emotional regulation behaviors are centered on these six emotional management maneuvers. A brief description of each of these methods is as follows.

Cognitive Reframing. Cognitive reframing centers on identifying and replacing distorted thinking with realistic and productive thoughts and beliefs. In this way the client can learn to generate adaptive emotional states by changing the nature of their cognitions. In other words, changing how we think in order to change the way we feel. An example of reframing is to substitute polarized thinking with more realistic and balanced thinking. The end result is to increase feelings that are less destructive and more positive, which is to say: hopeful, constructive, and fair/balanced.

Non-attachment. The practice of non-attachment is centered on letting go of one's emotions, sensations, and thoughts as they arise and without judgment. Feelings are not to be disengaged from or pushed away; rather, they are allowed to come into awareness and change from one moment to the next. In this case we take on the role of objective observer watching our feelings passing by like clouds drifting across a vast and luminous sky.

Accelerated Emotional Integration (AEI). AEI combines mindfulness with unconditional acceptance to return challenging emotions back into the overall energy of the mind. The end result of AEI is to naturalize otherwise harmful emotions. The analogy here is that of the wave (emotion) that melts back into the ocean (the mind) of which it is already a part.

Emotional Refinement. This is a more advanced form of emotional regulation that is based on Tibetan Buddhist tantric meditation. With emotional refinement, challenging emotions are refined into their positive state, e.g., anger into determination, fear into awareness, and sadness into compassion for others, etc. This method utilizes mindfulness, unconditional acceptance, and reframing in the service of unblocking emotional energy and allowing it to support a healthy and adaptive purpose. "The last way, which is also the riskiest, consists not in neutralizing emotions or looking into their void nature, but in transforming them, using them as catalysts for swiftly freeing oneself from their influence" (Goleman, 2003, p. 82).

Emotional Redirection. The redirection or channeling (sublimation) of emotional energy is one of consciously sublimating feelings into productive activities. Examples of this are physical exercise, creative pursuits, performing simple tasks such as house or yard work, and journaling about one's feelings.

Paradoxical Intentionality (PI). Paradoxical intentionality is the practice of simply doing the opposite of what one feels like doing in any given situation. Examples include willing one's self to get out of bed when one is depressed; acting with courage when one feels afraid; or acting with forgiveness or tolerance when one is angry. Paradoxical intentionality has much in common with behavioral exposure therapy and exposure with response prevention. By employing PI the patient can retrain their nervous system to be less reactive to aversive stimuli. On a more profound level PI can be utilized to promote deeper cognitive restructuring. Using PI to aid in achieving cognitive restructuring involves raising a client's affective state within the therapeutic environment. Once having done so, the patient is encouraged to tell their problem story as a means to bring to light unconscious core beliefs. Having raised these beliefs to the level of conscious awareness, the patient can be guided to challenge them by deliberately embracing their opposite (and more realistic) formulations.

Much can be written about each of these emotional management maneuvers; but for now it is sufficient to understand that, in order for a patient to safely master these methods, both group and individual therapy is recommended. The reason for this is that when working with emotions directly a client will run up against their own deeply entrenched behavior patterns. It is at this point that the client is most likely to encounter their resistance to change. Challenging deep seated maladaptive beliefs and behaviors must be balanced with kindness and compassion. The patient must be led to change by learning to be kind to themselves in their journey. Therefore, it is best to teach the APT emotional management practices in the overall context of the four APT coping modules rather than in a piecemeal fashion. This will better ensure a balanced approach to learning emotional regulation.

In the same manner, when teaching the skill of Direct Experiential Realization (DER) from the Insight/Mindfulness module, the therapist should make certain that the client is ready to see beyond their preconceived cognitive filters and assumptions about the self and reality. Like the advanced emotional regulation skills of emotional integration and emotional refinement, DER requires a profound shift in how a patient relates to their experiential input. Whether the client is experiencing a feeling, a thought, a mental object, or a bodily sensation, the skill of Direct Experiential Realization will challenge the client to engage their experience at a profoundly deeper, and more immediate level. Such experiential engagement can be threatening to even the most stable clients. Proceeding too quickly with DER can leave the client feeling overwhelmed by raw sensory input. A client who is unready to make such a shift with regard to their fundamental worldview may find themselves in the grip of powerful feelings of anxiety, and in some cases, existential dread. For this reason, the APT therapist must approach the teaching of DER with the certainty that the patient is well grounded in the APT coping skills. Likewise, the APT therapist must be sure that the client has a strong grasp of the Process-Self perspective.

Direct Experiential Realization is arrived at by looking deeply at a given phenomenon from the perspective of mindfulness. In a therapeutic setting the therapist will discuss the difference between a mental label and the phenomenon that the label is intended to describe. In this way the client begins to allow for psychological space to enter between the mental label and the phenomenon. The next phase to teaching DER is to guide the client to have an experience of a specific phenomenon as being made of object and non-object aspects. This is done while the client is in a state of mindfulness meditation. An example might be that of a drinking cup. While the client is in a state of mindful meditation, the therapist will point out that the cup depends on the empty space within the cup for it to exist as a receptacle for liquids. Without the empty space within the cup it would be a solid mass of ceramic. The therapist will then direct the client to notice additional non-cup elements such as the space surrounding the cup. Without the space surrounding the cup it could not exist as a container. The client could then be instructed to observe the shadow of the cup and the texture of the cup. The client might also be instructed to consider the many people and steps that went into the creation of the cup. The therapist would then instruct the client to notice the mental word "cup" as being superimposed over the cup-phenomenon. The mental object of a cup along with the thought "cup" would be let go of as the therapist instructs the client to recite the words: "this is a cup; this is a not-cup," or "cup; not-cup." The ultimate goal would be for the client to remain in mindfulness with single-pointed focus on a particular phenomenon until the client achieves an experience of the process-nature of the phenomenon. It is this direct experience beyond labels that is referred to as Suchness or Signlessness in Buddhism. "The greatest relief is when we break through the barriers of sign [cognitive labels] and touch the world of signlessness, nirvana" (Hanh, 1998, p. 149). The therapeutic benefit of breaking through one's mental labels to apprehend reality directly lies in deep cognitive restructuring. If a given phenomenon can be experienced as free flowing and empty of a fixed Object-Self nature, then all phenomena can be experienced as pure, free flowing *beingness* – including ourselves. It is the free flowing nature of *beingness* that best describes the integration of the Object-Self with the Process-Self perspective. From this integration it is possible for suffering to be transformed into the mind of wisdom, compassion, peace, and joy.

Chapter Six
The Cross Dialectic

*"We're only particles of change orbiting around the sun. But
how can I have that point of view when I'm always bound
and tied to someone" – Joni Mitchell*

The Layperson's Perspective

Doug Kraft, meditation teacher and author of Buddha's Map: His
Original Teachings on Awakening, Ease, and Insight in the Heart of
Meditation, writes of the importance of achieving a balance between
ease and effort in meditation. To assist a student in finding this
balance he recommends using what he calls the Six Rs of meditation:
Recognizing when the mind has become distracted; Releasing the
distraction; Relaxing any residual mental tension caused by the
distraction; Re-engaging one's smile (very important!); Returning to
the focus of your meditation such as the passage of air in and out of
your nostrils; and finally Radiating *metta* or the feeling of
friendliness like a candle that emits a warm glow of light in all
directions. If the meditator's mind becomes completely distracted by
some interesting mental object or mental script, the meditator can use
the Six Rs to gently return to a state of relaxed focus and mindfulness.
Of course, a beginning meditator's mind will tend to wander a great
deal. If she were to use the Six Rs every time she lost her focus she
would spend her entire time in meditation going over the Six Rs.
Instead, all that is required is to use the Six Rs only when the mind
has completely shifted into a state of distraction. The important thing
is to practice letting go of mental judgments that keep us from
uncovering our deeper mind of serenity and loving kindness. The Six
Rs offer us a powerful method by way of substituting a healthy
cognitive-behavioral script in place of negative, unwholesome
scripts.

From the standpoint of the Cross Dialectic, the Six Rs can serve
as an example of how we can segue from mental distraction by using

step one of the Cross Dialectic. Step one is that of unconditional acceptance. In acceptance we recognize and accept those things in life that we cannot change. This is also the first and second R (Recognize and Release) in the sequence of the Six Rs. Here we are noticing that our concentration has completely shifted to an object of distraction and then gently releasing the object. Step two in the Cross Dialect corresponds to the Relax, Re-engage your smile, Return to the object of your meditation, and Radiate the feeling of loving kindness in the Six Rs. In Step two of the Cross Dialect we find solutions for those aspects of the problem that we can change. In terms of meditation we can relax the mental tension of grasping or resisting. A good way to do this is to picture the tension as a wave in the ocean that melts back into the water. But any way that you can integrate the mental tension will work. The important thing to remember is that relaxing is a form of activity. We are doing something by relaxing our grip on the will to control. The next R in the sequence is to Re-engage your smile. When we smile we release endorphins and other neurotransmitters that give us a slight feeling of wellbeing. We are also changing our psychological state in the process. Finally, we gently return to the object of our meditation that we are using to help our mind to be centered in-the-moment. It is here that we can use the metaphor of the candle flame that gently Radiates warmth and light (*metta*) without any effort.

In steps three and four of the Cross Dialect we practice the steps of the sequence. By rehearsing the steps of the sequence we come into the flow of consciousness aspects of meditation. Practice, in Buddhism, depends on Right Effort. Right Effort refers to a relaxed but sustained effort as opposed to a forced effort. The Buddha used the example of the string of a lute to explain Right Effort to his students. If the lute string is too tight it produces a sharp note. If it is too lax it produces a flat note. Therefore, a balance of tension and ease is required when tuning the lute to produce a harmonious note. In steps three and four of the Cross Dialect we run through the sequence of the steps – using Right Effort – until they become natural. In terms of the Six Rs we run through the six steps until we no longer have to think about them. We have integrated the script to the point of becoming an unconscious habit. It is at this stage that we enter into a state of psychological flow (step four of the Cross Dialect).

We develop cognitive-behavioral scripts very early in life. They serve to help us make sense of the world and to save us time and energy. Our lives would be very difficult if we had to think about every step it takes to tie our shoes or take a sip of water. Fortunately, the human mind is capable of performing many tasks on autopilot. Problems arise when our ability to automate thinking and behaviors results in suffering. Habits can work for or against us depending on our own awareness of our internal scripts. If our habitual scripts compel us to act out in ways that produce feelings of anger, sadness, or worry, then we need to drop or modify our scripts. Those scripts that promote health and insight should be encouraged. In either case, our cognitive scripts should be seen as empty patterns of energy that ceaselessly come and go. They are like water in a stream or clouds in the sky. They have no abiding substance and can only cause us problems to the degree that we invest in them. But with mindfulness we can learn to let go of our attachment to our scripts. The practice of mindfully watching our scripts can lead to a greater ability to alter them for the better. A central goal of APT is to help a client to combine the skills of acceptance and positive change with sequencing and flow (the Cross Dialect). By learning to take charge of cognitive-behavioral scripts using such methods as the Cross Dialect, the Six Rs, and mindfulness, we can become increasingly empowered to shift into the Process-Self perspective. It is from the vantage of the Process-Self that we have the most freedom and ease regarding how we respond to life's many challenges.

The Clinical Perspective

The term "dialectics" refers to a connection between two polarized positions that have the potential to create a creative tension leading to a new dialectic. Friedrich Hegel, one of the original founders of dialectics and a major leader in German idealism, argued that, "The connection [between polar opposites] is of such a kind that any category, if scrutinized with sufficient care and attention, is found to lead to another" (McTaggart, 1986, p.1). Hegel identified three fundamental positions that he defined as thesis and antithesis on either extreme that can result in a creative synthesis. An example of this is going to a car dealership and being offered three choices: a black car, a white car, or some variation of a grey car. However, if we combine the best aspects of black and white we can come up with the entire spectrum of color possibilities for a new car. We do not have to settle for black, white, or grey. For Auto Process Therapy, the *thesis* equals self, the *antithesis* equals no-self, which leads to the *synthesis* of the thesis and antithesis. In this equation, self plus no-self combines to generate the Process-Self (self + no-self = Process-Self).

Without getting into a detailed discussion on the philosophical underpinning of dialectical theory, it is enough to understand that people often find themselves caught on the proverbial horns of a dilemma. With regard to the patient's emotional experience, the dilemma often plays out in the form of fight, flight, or freeze. Therefore, a central aim of APT is to teach a patient how to resolve dilemmas and thus begin to move forward where once they experienced paralysis. To this end the cross dialectic therapeutic maneuver comes into play.

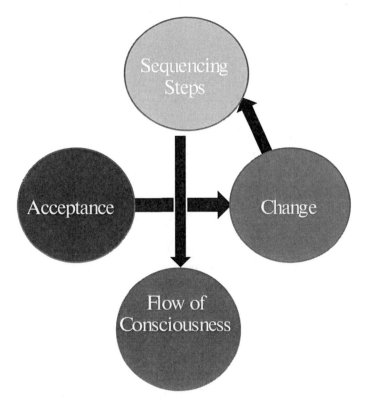

Figure 1.

The cross dialectic maneuver provides a sequence of four steps that begins on the horizontal axis with *unconditional acceptance*, moving to *effective change*, and continues to *sequencing steps* and finally *flow of consciousness* on the vertical axis (Figure 1). The area on the horizontal axis between "radical acceptance" and effective change forms the foundation of Dialectical Behavioral Therapy (DBT) as conceived by Marsha Linehan (Marra, 2005, p. 109). Linehan defines radical acceptance as a "turning of the mind," *unconditionally*, to acceptance in-the-moment (Linehan, 1993, p. 176). The rationale for teaching a patient to endure strong feelings versus venting them is that acting on toxic emotions only increases destructive behavioral reactivity. "Besides increasing emotionality directly, inappropriate, mood-dependent behavior usually leads to consequences that elicit other unwanted emotions" (Linehan, 1993, p. 46). In regards to APT, the core of unconditional acceptance is to develop a willingness to experientially confront one's deepest fears, not the least of which is fear of death. "If we know the reality of no birth and no death [selflessness], we can transcend all fear" (Hanh, 2006, p. 37). Unconditional acceptance (step one on the cross dialectic maneuver) depends upon making a choice to courageously return one's awareness to the here-and-now, even when our current experience is painful or unpleasant. The other key component to unconditional acceptance is cognitive reframing. A cognitive reframe is choosing to view something in a positive light such as seeing the glass as half full versus half empty. So these two skills, unconditional experiential awareness along with cognitive reframing, combine to create a state of free flowing psychological acceptance.

On the other side of the dialectic, effective change speaks to assuming a solution oriented perspective in one's current circumstances (step two on the cross dialectic maneuver). Solutions cannot be put into place in the past or the future. Although it is useful to plan ahead, as well as to reflect on the errors of the past, the solution focused approach remains firmly rooted in the present. When we put these two together, unconditional acceptance and effective change, we naturally arrive at their synthesis, creative solutions.

Once a solution is recognized, the next position on the cross dialectic (step three on the cross dialectic maneuver) is to break down the solution into a sequence of manageable steps. Sequencing a problem allows a patient to practice a procedure until it becomes a more natural process. The vertical axis of the cross dialect refers to procedural knowledge. Lastly, step four on the cross dialectic maneuver refers to process knowledge that leads to a state of flow. "Your mind isn't wandering, you are not thinking of something else; you are totally involved in what you are doing" (Csikszentmihalyi, 1990, p. 53). The bridge between content knowledge in which we sequence the steps of the dance, and process knowledge in which we surrender to the flow of the dance, is achieved through the utilization of practice and repetition.

To illustrate how one might apply the cross dialect maneuver to the problem of obesity (step one on the cross dialectic) the patient would first attempt to unconditionally accept the condition of being overweight. In this example being overweight is a fact. To deny this fact is to delude oneself (denial). Unconditional acceptance is not a judgment about one's character, but rather, an objective observation.

From this perspective the patient can then move to an effective change position (step two) on the cross dialectic. It is here that the patient might conclude that a diet and exercise program is in order. However, rather than plunge headfirst into an unrealistic regime of exercise and diet, a sensible plan needs to be established. Planning takes us to step three where the patient would outline the phases of diet and exercise from the earlier stages of treatment and apply them to this middle stage of treatment. Finally, having worked out the steps of the solution the patient would then act on the plan (step four). It is here that Paradoxical Intentionality or doing the opposite of what we feel like doing, can be applied. Merely thinking about jumping on the long ignored treadmill in the spare bedroom is not enough. Until we act on our intentions by applying consistent effort our healthy intentions do us little good. Along with positive intention and consistent effort, it is vital to develop new habits, acting through practice, and establishing a new internal rhythm. In Buddhist terms this is what is referred to as internal karma or habit energy. Once the nervous system becomes habituated to exercise it begins to crave it. Now we are in the flow of the behavior and no longer need to force ourselves to exercise.

Another common life challenge people encounter is the difficult person. When we encounter the difficult person in our lives we typically default to anger and judgment. But such a reaction is only self-reinforcing. However, by applying the cross dialectic to the situation we can defuse a problem before it begins. Again, we start by unconditionally accepting the fact that we cannot control the actions of another human being (step one). Nor can we expect other people to share our values or our personal sensibilities about appropriate conduct. Having accepted the fact that we cannot control the behavior of others, the next step is to consider what we *can* change about the situation (step two). Often the very thing that we can change is how we respond to the difficult person. It is at this point that our communication behaviors and ethical behaviors come to the fore. Effective communication is honest and congruent with our values and principles. Likewise this is so with effective actions. It is often the case when dealing with difficult people that we must simply maintain our position using a broken record approach. As long as we remain objective and non-judgmental we can assert our position without resorting to verbal attacks. At this stage we are ready to plan our sequence of responsive behaviors, and finally, put them into action (step three). Difficult people are typically highly emotional and irrational. This state makes them egocentric as well. For this reason it can be advantageous for us to remain mindful and counter their high emotionality with reason, calm, and kindness. This approach has the effect of calming the other person's extreme emotionality. However, we must also be mindful that the difficult person may escalate in emotionality before returning to a more balanced state of mind. For this reason it is sometimes necessary to remove oneself from their physical proximity. In extreme cases the intervention of law enforcement might be the only safe course of action.

Returning to step four, flow of consciousness, the state of flow is characterized by the qualities of ease and awareness. However, in the beginning phase of flow it is common to trend towards unconscious, habitual behavior while performing the sequence of steps in the process. Many people are satisfied to remain uninvolved in the task at hand provided they do not slip up. Everyone has had the experience of arriving at work without any memory of having actually driven there. However, one of the meta-goals of APT is objective awareness in-the-moment; a state of mind more commonly referred to as mindfulness. This being the case, the second phase of step four of the cross dialectic is characterized by a loss of self-consciousness leading to the state of flow. When not preoccupied with ourselves, we actually have a chance to expand the concept of who we are. Loss of self-consciousness can lead to self-transcendence, to a feeling that the boundaries of our being have been pushed forward." (Csikszentmihalyi, 1990, p. 53). It is this loss of self-as-object leading to self-transcendence that is a defining characteristic of the Process-Self perspective. At this stage of treatment the patient begins to access deeper levels of being. It is at stage four that a shift in perspective is possible, from the reactive Object-Self, to the more adaptive and responsive Process-Self.

A summary of the four steps of the Cross Dialectic

- **Unconditional Acceptance.** Unconditional acceptance of things as they are using positive reframing and mindfulness in tandem.

- **Positive Mindset.** Focus on solutions rather than problems. Do not get caught up in the problems of the past or future. Do not get caught up in cognitive-behavioral patterns of negativity.

- **Sequence the Solution.** Break the solution into manageable steps and lay them out in a logical order from start to finish.

- **Implementation and Integration.** Practice the sequence of the steps to the solution until the scr

Chapter Seven
The Meta-cognitive Reprocessing Maneuver

*"Let the wise man guard his thoughts, for they are
difficult to perceive, very artful, and they rush
wherever they want"* — The Dhammapada

The Layperson's Perspective

Reality is an ongoing energetic process. It is the ultimate nature of
reality that it has neither an inside nor an outside. This is to say that
reality is all of one cloth. It is only Man that makes a distinction
between an inner reality and an outer one. Within the realm of energy
such distinctions are fuzzy at best. All that we can say with any
degree of certainty is that the energy of the universe can exist in either
a potential or an active state. When energy manifests in its active
mode it is in a constant process of change. When it is in a potential
state it exists as pure abstraction – a hypothetical unit of force – that
has yet to become exhibited within an energy system. According to
Buddhist psychology, energy that is in its dormant state is like a seed
(*bija*) that is hidden in our unconscious mind. The seed only waits to
be watered by our attachments to become the active expressions of
energy. Once the seed is activated its energy plays out in the form of
a mental script. Along with the mental script there is an associated
emotional charge. The interaction between attachment, seed, and
mental script describes the activity of *samskara* or habit energy. Over
time the script becomes a part of our self-identity and thus our
attachment grows even stronger. As our attachments grow, so does
our sense of craving. It is craving that is the primary form of suffering
from which all other forms of mental anguish arise. Liberation from
suffering, therefore, depends upon replacing our attachment to
mental scripts that obscure our view of reality. By gradually learning
to let go of our mental scripts we can begin to experience an
underlying formless reality of equanimity and love.

Our mental scripts run through our mind twenty-four hours a day, seven days a week. For the most part they operate in the background and serve a useful purpose. The downside of this arrangement is that we tend to go through life in a kind of hypnotic trance. We are so swayed by the force of our scripts that we rarely question the representation of reality that our scripts present to us. Caught up in a dualistic worldview, we seem to be moving through life on a narrow path from past to future. From our mistaken point of view the universe is outside of us and within us is the mind. Somewhere deep in the mind we sense a unique self that seems to represent the essence of who we are. Much of our energy goes into defending this self against pain and annihilation. But in our efforts to maintain the integrity of the self we widen the divide between the inner world and the outer. In the end we lose all touch with core awareness that is at the heart of reality.

A central therapeutic maneuver of APT is the Meta-cognitive Reprocessing Maneuver or RM. The RM is designed to guide a client through the stages of detachment to non-attachment. Understanding the role of attachment or *tanha* (thirst) is central to the practical application of Buddhism. It is *tanha* that takes a simple desire and degrades it into a state of craving or addictive obsession. There is a story in Japanese Zen Buddhism that illustrates the process by which we turn a natural desire into the suffering of craving. In the story, two Buddhist monks were returning to their monastery by way of a forest path in the woods. As they walked together in mindfulness they encountered a geisha girl standing at the bank of a wide stream. "Please," the geisha asked the two monks as they approached, "can one of you carry me across the stream so that I don't ruin my kimono by getting it wet?" The older monk replied that he would happily carry her across the stream and proceeded to gather her up in his arms. All the while the geisha and the monk laughed and flirted as men and women will sometimes do. Upon reaching the other side of the stream the monk put the geisha down and the two parted company. The two monks continued on their way in silence. However, the younger monk was at war with himself the entire time. He was at a loss to understand how his venerable brother could defile himself by touching such a woman! After all, had he not taken a vow to shun all sexual and romantic contact with the opposite sex? And yet, here he was laughing and flirting with this woman. He even carried her in his arms across the stream! At last the younger monk could stand it no longer and he exclaimed, "How could you break your vow of chastity and touch that woman?" But the older monk, surprised by the younger monk's outburst, replied, "Are you still carrying her around? I put her down two hours ago."

This story illustrates the difference between desire, which is a natural and necessary element of the human experience, and attachment. The older monk had no shame or guilt concerning his attraction to the beautiful geisha girl. His sexual desire was a natural and healthy response to her. However, unlike the younger monk, he was non-attached to his desire. As soon as he parted company with the geisha he shifted his focus to mindfully walking in the forest. The younger monk, by contrast, was not only attached to his repressed sexual desire, he was also attached to his feelings of shame and guilt about his sexual desire. The end result was to propel him into a state of consternation about the actions of the older monk. Had the younger monk mentally put the girl down at the edge of the stream he would not have experienced self-induced suffering. He would have been non-attached to his sexual attraction and so let it integrate naturally into the totality of his mind. It is the practice of cultivating non-attachment to our desires that best describes the method of Buddhist mindfulness meditation or *vipassana*.

The RM depends on the client making a shift from attachment to the problem story, and into a state on non-attachment. From the standpoint of non-attachment we can gain the overview perspective. From the overview we can observe our mental scripts from a safe distance, metaphorically speaking. We can look down on the interesting features of the mind without generating more attachment. The particulars of our mental scripts can be examined from a new vantage point. The various features of the mental scripts such as colors, textures, images, and sensations can be identified. The power of the mental script fades as the component parts are deconstructed. Finally, after progressing from detachment to non-attachment, we are ready to make the descent back into our sense of physical form. Our mind is open to the experience of core awareness or what in Buddhism is referred to as Buddha Nature. The grip of *tanha* has been relaxed and we can open ourselves to the gentle but powerful voice of our deeper, innate intelligence. The experience is like the sudden realization that we have a solution to a vexing problem. We have slept on it and then, through no particular effort on our part, the answer simply pops into our awareness. We laugh at how we struggled over such an obvious solution. The answer had been there all along! But, because of our craving for control, we pushed it away. Now, in the relaxed and open space of mindful non-attachment, the solution reveals itself.

The Clinical Perspective

In recent years much has been made of the cultivation of mindfulness as a therapeutic practice. "Although mindfulness meditation was originally developed in the Buddhist religious tradition, it has been adopted by Western psychology as a nonreligious strategy to decrease emotional suffering" (Marra, 2005, p. 22). It is also fair to say that mindfulness does play a significant role in the practical day-to-day application of Buddhism. As one of the insight behavioral skills, mindfulness combines one-pointedness with non-judgment in the Noble Eightfold Path. Without a doubt, mindfulness, as defined as objective global awareness in-the-moment, is a critical element to the practice of Zazen and other forms of Buddhist meditation. In APT, it is the central aim of mindfulness practice to cultivate a state of non-attachment from obsessive pleasure seeking (addiction), aggression and pain avoidance (resistance), and ignorance (unconsciousness/denial). Another important application of the mindfulness behavioral coping skill is to serve as a psychological impartial space from which to transition into other coping behaviors. In his book, Eight Mindful Steps to Happiness, Henepola Gunaratana points out that mindfulness is analogous to shifting into a neutral gear in order to transition into other gears. With regard to APT, the practice of mindfulness is utilized to facilitate shifting into one of the APT therapeutic maneuvers. Chief among these is the Meta-cognitive Reprocessing Maneuver (RM).

A central aim of the RM is to help the client to distinguish between unconscious attachments on the one hand, and conscious non-attachment on the other. Non-attachment can be defined as consciously engaging in, while letting go of, thoughts, feelings, and sensations in-the-moment. As such, non-attachment needs to be clearly understood as being different from the psychological state of detachment. Furthermore, both detachment and non-attachment are understood as being unique states of mind that are distinct from the unconscious, pathological state of dissociation.

Psychological dissociation is the ego's attempt to protect the mind by repressing traumatic experiences and feelings. Dissociation is characterized by "a disruption of and/or discontinuity in the normal integration of consciousness, memory, identity, emotion, perception, body representation, motor control, and behavior" (American Psychiatric Association, 2013, p. 291). Dissociation, then, is defined as a pathological state of mind and is therefore destructive. By contrast, in the state of *detachment* the sense of self, while being fully aware of its current circumstances, becomes emotionally cut off from relationships and situations that would otherwise engage emotions. For the purpose of the reprocessing maneuver, conscious intentional detachment is used as a precursor to non-attachment in the service of resolving emotional distress.

A good way to explain the distinction between detachment and non-attachment is the metaphor of the stream bank. If we stand on the stream bank and watch the flowing water as it passes by, we are detached from the actual experience of the water. We understand that the stream is flowing before us. However, we have no emotional or experiential understanding of the nature of the water. Non-attachment takes our understanding one step further. In non-attachment we leave the safety of the stream bank and wade into the stream itself. Now we can feel the water as it swirls around our legs. We can see the river from the perspective of being in the middle of the stream. And yet, we do not allow ourselves to be swept away by the flowing waters. We are firmly rooted in the middle of the stream. All of which speaks to a conscious involvement on our part. The moment we slip into unawareness non-attachment is lost. As such, it runs counter to our efforts to realize the Process-Self perspective. It is for this reason that, in the practice of non-attachment, we strive to experience and accept both painful and pleasurable experiences without resistance or judgments. "A gardener does not chase after flowers and try to run away from garbage. She accepts both and she takes care of both" (Hanh, 2006, p.246).

We begin the reprocessing maneuver by summarizing the various issues the patient brings to the session into a single problem statement. This is stage one: problem summary, identification, and externalization. The goal is to reduce the patient's complex issues into a more manageable and resolvable challenge. Once the thought distortion or problem thought is singled out, it is then possible to create psychological distance between the patient's sense of self and the problem thought. The goal at this point is to externalize the thought as existing in the patient's life rather than being an inseparable part of the patient's core identity.

Stage 1: The breakdown in stage one

- Create a problem statement out of the patient's account of the various issues, e.g., "I feel like my life is out of control and I just can't get a handle on anything."
- Identify the main problem as a discrete problem thought – "My life is completely out of control."
- Externalize the problem thought – "I am a person with a feeling of being out of control that is dominating my life."

Having defined the problem statement and the problem thought along with successfully externalizing the problem, we proceed to stage two. In stage two the goal is to process the thoughts and the feelings in terms of their underlying meaning by using standard cognitive behavioral approaches. At this point we are analyzing cognitions in preparation for the reprocessing that will come in the final stages of the reprocessing maneuver. Stage two then consists of processing the thoughts and the feelings linked to the patient's problem story. The problem story is the narrative that the patient extrapolates out of the problem thought or thought distortion. The problem thought is a manifestation of the underlying maladaptive, unconscious schema. A schema, according to the theory of cognitive behavioral psychology, is the mixture of feelings, images, and beliefs that give rise to thought distortions. "Schemas are cognitive structures within the mind, the specific content of which are core beliefs" (Beck, 1995, p. 166).

Stage 2: Processing the thoughts and feelings associated with the Problem Story

- What do you *think* about this story including images and memories?
- How does this story make you *feel*?
- What does this story *mean* to you if it is true?

This brings us to stage three in which we detach from the problem story, the feelings linked to the story, and the meaning of the story. At this stage in the RM the client is assisted in consciously detaching from the various feelings and cognitions associated with the problem story. It is here that they can then begin to safely experience the psychological pain that often results from bringing their maladaptive schema into consciousness. However, it must be strongly noted that this maneuver can only be safely accomplished within the therapeutic milieu under the guidance of a skilled APT therapist. This is due to the need to increase a patient's affect in order to bring the underlying schema into full consciousness. The method then, of stage three, is to guide the patient in visualizing themselves as if they are floating above their mind from the standpoint of looking down. The various contents of the mind, thoughts, feelings, sensations, images, etc., are then simply labeled and assigned color, textures, weight, or any other suitable, symbolic appellation. The goal, at this stage, is to generate a state of detachment rather than to come to a resolution of the presenting issues.

Stage 3: Detachment (Meta-cognitive Perspective)

- Visualize yourself floating above the landscape of your mind.
- Label and describe your images, feelings, perceptions, and memories.
- Do they have a color, texture, or weight? Are they solid, liquid, or soft?

Lastly we come to stage four, the reprocessing phase. It is at this juncture that we can employ the imagery of the stream bank and the stream. If we have not already walked the patient through a guided imagery journey, then now would be an optimum time to do so. In this stage the goal is to teach the patient to gain the meta-cognitive overview of the situation. From this perspective the patient can at once experience and review the various aspects of his or her life in a holistic manner. It is here that the therapist must join with the patient during the non-attachment exercise. To this end, the appropriate use of countertransference is employed. The skillful APT therapist will shift into a state of mindful non-attachment, joining with the patient in a meditative state, and proceed to connect with his or her own deeper mind. In doing so, the therapist will open the way for unconscious material to surface into awareness. The therapist will then share (only *after* the patient has had a chance to first share) any thoughts, images, or perceptions that might have presented in meditation. However, the therapist will always run the risk of trading the role of counselor for that of client when making personal disclosures to a patient. For this reason the therapist must be able to justify, in therapeutic terms, his or her choice to share personal information. Therefore, at the end of stage four of the RM, sharing of any impressions that the therapist has during the meditation should be kept to a minimum. An example of an impression that the therapist might have could be, "I saw an image of a child under an apple tree when I was joining you in meditation just now. It made me feel peaceful. I wonder if that adds to your experience during the meditation." It is very possible that the therapist's impressions have no meaning for the patient. If so, the therapist will express casual acceptance and move on. Conversely, the therapist's impressions, which have been developed on an unconscious level during the session, may be of importance to the client and so spark further insights. The importance of following this format became clear to me when I first attempted the RM with a volunteer whom I shall refer to as Mary.

We attempted the Reprocessing Maneuver only after Mary had completed six weeks of an APT, life enhancement coach program. As it turned out, Mary proved to be an ideal student of APT due to her own extensive background in Buddhism. We began the session as if she were a first time client. Mary spent a good deal of time in phase one of the RM and I began to worry that we could not finish the entire maneuver in one hour. However, by redirecting Mary to sum up her thoughts into a simple problem statement, we were able to continue to the next phases. When we reached the detachment phase of the RM, Mary pointed out the risk that some clients might not be able to fully reconnect to their bodies. If an untrained therapist allowed them to remain with a sense of "floating above themselves" beyond the meditation the patient might slip into a harmful state of dissociation. I took this into consideration and made a mental note to emphasize that the client must not attempt the RM outside of the therapeutic milieu. At last we arrived at the non-attachment phase of the maneuver. I had been reading Jack Kornfield's The Wise Heart at the time and so, inspired by Kornfield's method of joining his clients in meditation, I went into a state of mindful non-attachment along with Mary. As I guided her to accept all thoughts, feelings, and sensations like water flowing through her being, I began to see a pink ball of light forming in the center of my field of vision. We sat in silence for a few minutes and then I asked Mary to share her impressions of the RM. She stated that her deeper mind had offered the word, "love," as the answer to her challenge. I told her of my own impressions of a pink light and feeling of unconditional love, which she said had fit with a meditation she had recently experienced. As we talked I realized the significance of this turn of events. By including my own countertransference into the process (after Mary had a chance to share) I was able to tap into a greater source of understanding than my academic, thinking mind could have offered. We agreed that the therapist should share his or her impression only after the client shares. In this way the client is not influenced by the countertransference of the therapist.

Stage 4: Reprocessing the underlying schema (from conscious detachment to non-attachment)

- Relax, breathe, and center.

- Allow all thoughts, feelings, and sensations associated with the schema to pass away like leaves floating down a stream.

- Focus completely on experiencing the flow of new thoughts, feelings, and sensations as they arise in-the-moment. Unconditionally accept them as they are, feeling them without clinging or rejecting.

- Re-orientate to the room by focusing on the bottom of your feet and the sensation of breathing. Come back to your sense of self in the room. Affirm: I am strong enough. I am loveable enough. I am worthy enough. **Therapist's countertransference**: having joined with the patient in meditation, share whatever thoughts, feelings, or perceptions came into your mind when you connected to your own deeper mind.

The overall goal of the reprocessing maneuver is to teach the patient to view any challenge from the perspective of non-attachment. From the standpoint of non-attachment the client is better disposed to have a recognition of their own deeper wisdom or Buddha Nature. By connecting with their Buddha Nature the patient can learn to access hidden internal resources. The actual resolution of a specific issue may or may not arise out of the reprocessing maneuver. In this way the reprocessing maneuver differs from cognitive-behavioral techniques. A central objective of cognitive-behavioral therapy is to identify and challenge maladaptive beliefs. The primary purpose of the reprocessing maneuver is to find resolution in mindful acceptance and non-attachment. The benefit of doing so is to ready the patient to make a shift from the grasping and rejecting Object-Self; and into the adaptive and resilient Process-Self. A crucial step leading to this goal is to teach the patient the concept of metacognition. The RM, by design, is meta-cognitive in nature. By guiding the patient through the four stages of the reprocessing maneuver the patient will gain an experience of adaptive, conscious detachment leading to non-attachment. From this perspective the patient will begin to gain the ability to rise above and allow for a broad range of emotionally charged experiences – painful or otherwise – without distress or cognitive impairment.

A summary of the stages of the reprocessing maneuver
Stage 1. Problem summary

- Create a problem statement out of the patient's account of the various issues, e.g., "I feel like my life is out of control and I just can't get a handle on anything."
- Identify the main problem as a discrete problem thought – "My life is completely out of control."
- Externalize the problem thought – "I am a person with a feeling of being out of control that is dominating my life."

Stage 2. Cognitive Processing, Developing Non-Identification

- What do you *think* about this story including images and memories?
- How does this story make you *feel*? What does this story *mean* to you if it is true?

Stage 3. Detachment from the schema (Meta-cognitive Perspective)

- Visualize yourself floating above the landscape of your mind.
- Label and describe your images, feelings, perceptions, and memories. Do they have a color, texture, or weight? Are they solid, liquid, or soft?

Stage 4. Non-Attachment and Integration

- Relax, breathe, and center.

- Allow all thoughts, feelings, and sensations associated with the schema to pass away like leaves floating downstream.

- Focus completely on experiencing the flow of new thoughts, feelings, and sensations as they arise in-the-moment and unconditionally accept them as they are; feeling them without clinging or rejecting.

- Re-orientate to the room by focusing on the bottom of your feet and the sensation of breathing. Come back to your sense of self in the room. Affirm: I am strong enough. I am loveable enough. I am worthy enough. I feel good about who I am. **Therapist's countertransference**: Having joined with the patient in meditation, share whatever thoughts, feelings, or perceptions came into your mind when you connected to your own deeper mind.

Chapter Eight
The Four Behavioral Skills Modules and The APT Diary Card

*"And this, monks, is the noble truth of the path
leading to the cessation of suffering;
just this Noble Eightfold Way"* — Gautama Buddha

The Layperson's Perspective

When the Object-Self is removed what remains is a continuing state of awakening. Awakening is not the same as having a fixed and unchanging self. There is no actual self within the state of awakening. Rather, awakening comprehends a selfless, core awareness that radiates infinite intelligence and boundless compassion. Who then becomes awakened? The simple answer is that we do. The entire person-in-process is the one who becomes awakened to core awareness. This is what the Buddha meant when he described himself as the *Tathagate* or the one who is continually coming from suchness (the absolute, process nature of reality) and returning to suchness. The real question is: what is it that is keeping us in a state of unconsciousness? The answer lies in understanding the relationship between intentional actions and outcomes. This relationship is what is understood in Buddhism as karma.

Buddhism outlines a series of psychological events that begins with ignorance and ends with suffering. This series of events is called the twelve link chain of dependent origination (of suffering and rebirth). The chain of dependent origination represents an in-depth model of the entire mind-stream. The first "link" in the chain refers to ignorance (*avijja*) of the selfless, process nature of reality. Because we believe that we exist as solid and separate entities in a world of discrete objects, we operate in a state of fundamental misunderstanding or ignorance. However, this state of affairs is not the same as a conceptual misunderstanding of reality. The conceptual manifestation of *avijja* comes at the end of the chain of mind moments. *Avijja* refers to an inherent tendency to be blind to the process nature of things. It is like being born color blind or deaf. For purposes of survival we simply are not equipped by nature to be predisposed to arriving at the Process-Self perspective. Our inherent bias towards an Object-Self perspective gives rise to a host of thinking errors and delusions. Furthermore, our delusions are reinforced by society and culture from a very early age. In addition, there is the need for children to solve a variety of development tasks designed to reinforce a healthy ego function. Add to this the power of deeply entrenched, conditioned behavioral habits and the foundation of delusion is firmly established.

The Buddha outlined a specific path designed to counteract the conditioning that prevents us from awakening to the true nature of reality. From the standpoint of psychotherapy the Buddha's eightfold path falls into the category of cognitive behavioral interventions. The eight aspects of the path are: right views or accurate understanding of reality; right intentions or thinking; right speech or communication; right actions or conduct; right occupation or livelihood; right or balanced effort; right mindfulness; and right concentration. "Right" can be interpreted as being wise, effective, and leading to harmonious outcomes. Auto Process Therapy expands on the noble eightfold path by breaking it down into specific coping behaviors. The list of APT coping behaviors is grouped into four domains: discernment or thinking behaviors; ethical action behaviors; insight or mindfulness behaviors; and *bodhichitta* or emotional management behaviors.

One of the main points that the APT behavioral coping skills are designed to convey is the importance of linking behavior with feelings. Tanha or craving – which is the primary driver of suffering – arises out of ignorance. Ignorance, in this sense, refers to our natural bias towards thinking in terms of our own self-interest. Tanha, then, is the tension that arises from the perceptual splint between self and other. In a physical sense tanha manifests as neurological tension. It also takes on the characteristic of psychological tension in the form of grasping as the self reaches out to possess the object of desire. For the purposes of APT, grasping is understood to be an internal behavior that generates painful emotions. When we bend our will to obtain the object of desire we are investing in an internal behavior. The more we invest in grasping behavior the more we generate feelings of frustration, anger, fear, sadness, or self-pity. Even when we manage to temporarily obtain that which we are grasping for we are not satisfied. The emotional high of getting what we want soon fades as all emotions must. This is the meaning of dukkha or the suffering that results from the inevitable dissatisfaction of obtaining our desires. Dukkha prompts us reach out yet again for next desirable thing. On and on this cycle goes, churning out disappointment and frustration. And because we fail to understand the role of grasping in the cycle of suffering, we repeat the same habitual patterns indefinitely. The interaction of grasping and suffering, therefore, is the energy that fuels the entire apparatus of suffering.

On an intuitive level we tend to assume that, because we feel something, we are driven to react in order to satisfy that feeling. I sense that I am hungry, and the emotion of desire arises in my mind. I then seek out a snack to fulfill my desire and end my hunger. But if we look more closely with the eyes of mindfulness we can see that we have overlooked a critical step. Between the sensory input from the body and our decision to find food there is a subtle, non-verbal attachment at work. Even before we can articulate the conscious thought, "I want something to eat," we are unconsciously reaching out to take hold of the desired object. It is at this point that we engage in the internal behavior of grasping. The choice to grasp – which is an internal, mental action – gives rise to an emotion. In this case, the emotion of desire arises in response to the habit of attaching to not wanting to feel hungry. Following this chain of events to its logical conclusion, we might soon find ourselves in search of the nearest fast food restaurant. The act of seeking out a fast food restaurant serves to reinforce the subtle attachment to junk food.

As a therapeutic goal, APT aims to provide clients with a variety of behavioral replacement strategies. These strategies are designed to afford a client with a degree of behavioral leverage over their moods and emotions. An example might be using the discernment skill of "checking the facts" before assuming to know why another motorist has suddenly entered the lane in front of us. Our internal habit script might kick in and play out a sequence of mental events in which we are being discounted by the other driver. However, if we stop to challenge this mental script with the facts of the matter, we might notice that the driver was simply trying to avoid a road hazard. There was no deliberate intention to display disrespect by suddenly changing lanes.

Even before we check the facts we can practice the skill of emotional integration. Let us use the example of the unpredictable motorist once again. In this situation it might be helpful to first let the feeling of anger melt back into the neutral state of pure awareness. From the stance of mindful acceptance, we watch as the feeling of anger rises like a wave in our mind-body complex. The anger/wave abides for a moment and floods our body with neurotransmitters to prep us for fight, flight, or freeze. We notice, from the vantage point of centering on our breath, that the anger/wave is now melting into the overall totality of the mind. We feel a sense of relief and even humor as the energy of the wave dissipates. In its place other waves of emotional energy arise in an endless parade of feeling. We are mindful of the mental script that accompanied the anger/wave as well. It too has subsided. We have returned to a relaxed state of process and are ready to challenge our assumptions by checking the facts. We might also employ the skills of being grateful or of self-soothing by listening to music on our car radio. Using humor and kindness (*metta*) we avoid the pitfall of grasping at *not* grasping. We notice the mental self-object of the "enlightened" person rising up in our mind, and we smile. This is a trap that we have learned to sidestep with gentleness and playful awareness. We know better than to invest in grasping at being the kind of person who does not grasp. By using the skill-set of the Six Rs we quickly return to the here-and-now. Throughout it all we remember to use the skill of having a "workmanlike attitude" by focusing on progress, not perfection. We are in a calm and receptive state in which there is space for any number of insights and positive feelings to emerge. They bob to the surface, in a manner of speaking, without any effort on our part. These are the seeds of enlightenment that are buried deep within our store consciousness. They have been there all along. But, because of our attachment to ego and power, we have been unable to take full advantage of them. Now, as we learn to shift into the free flowing state of process, we can rest assured that we already possess the internal resources required to be happy and at ease. We can begin to abandon our "coping skills" and embrace life enhancing maneuvers. It is at this point that we can make the shift from survive to thrive.

The Clinical Perspective

Just as it is unlikely that an inexperienced climber will reach the top of a high mountain without a guide, so the patient is also unlikely to achieve the Process-Self perspective without a coherent path to follow. In this chapter I will outline such a path as well as the APT diary cards. It is through the application of the diary cards that the various APT behavioral coping skills are acquired.

In my experience most clients are intellectually capable of understanding the concept of Object-Self versus Process-Self. However, this understanding remains only a philosophical exercise without achieving a deep cognitive restructuring of the self-schema. This being stated, in order to safely facilitate cognitive restructuring without increasing the patient's emotional distress it is essential to master the behavioral skills that comprise the four coping behaviors modules of APT. Central to mastering the four modules is the APT diary card.

The APT diary card allows the patient to familiarize him or herself with, integrate, and embody, the APT behavioral skills on a daily basis. By making use of the diary card the patient can then report their progress, as well as their setbacks, to the therapist in both an individual and group setting. In this way the patient is able to increase his or her confidence in their ability to cope with distressful feelings. It cannot be emphasized enough that a sense of emotional efficacy is critical to gaining a stable identity. In the absence of a solid sense of self it is not possible to establish a general state of equanimity. As paradoxical as it may sound given that APT argues attachment to the self is the primary cause of anguish, one must have a strong ego-function in order to transcend the ego. Only by learning to see past the ego-function – while still maintaining its activity of regulating psychic energy – can we enter into a state of pure, selfless process beyond grasping and aversion. It is through self-transcendence that we can at last choose between suffering and ease.

> The 'I' concept is a process. It is something we are constantly doing. With vipassana (mindfulness meditation) we learn to see that we are doing it, when we are doing it, and how we are doing it. Then that mindset moves and fades away, like a cloud passing through a sky.
>
> (Gunarantana, 2011, p. 32).

Use of the diary card also allows the therapist to monitor the patient's progress and for the other group members to offer feedback to the patient. The diary card encourages the patient to be honest about the amount of time and effort that they are actually putting into learning APT. It is imperative, however, that the patient is not made to feel invalidated should they neglect the daily discipline of using the diary cards. If it comes out in therapy that the patient is resistant to using the diary cards this becomes an opportunity to practice the behavioral skill of paradoxical intentionality. "Behavioral-expressive responses are important parts of all emotions. Thus one strategy to change or regulate an emotion is to change its behavioral-expressive component by acting in a way that opposes or is inconsistent with the emotions" (Linehan, 1993, p. 85).

With regard to the four behavioral coping skills modules, i.e., *prajna*/discernment skills, *karma*/ethical action/skills, *samadhi*/insight skills, and *bodhichitta*/compassion skills, the core competencies related to each of the modules are derived directly from the Buddha's Noble Eightfold Path. The Noble Eightfold Path is the Buddhist program of moral and ethical development leading to a deepening understanding of self and reality. The ultimate goal of the Noble Eightfold Path is the extinction of suffering and the attainment of enlightenment. Enlightenment, although difficult to define, can be understood as being an experiential awakening to the selfness, process nature of reality:

"This, O Monks, is the Noble Truth of the Path which leads to the cessation of suffering: that holy Eightfold Path, that is to say, Right Belief, Right Aspiration, Right Speech, Right Conduct, Right Means of Livelihood, Right Endeavor, Right Mindfulness, Right Meditation" (Noss, 1999, p. 175).

The Buddha did not specify in detail what any of the aspects of the path entailed. Nonetheless, he was clear that adherence to the path results in positive outcomes and a decrease in suffering. It is, therefore, up to the individual to decide what the various facets of the path are for themselves.

The Noble Eightfold Path is divided into three general areas designed to build one upon the other: *prajna*/discriminating wisdom, *sila*/ethical and moral action, and *samadhi*/insight (Noss, 1987). Borrowing a page from Marsha Linehan's dialectical behavioral therapy, I have added an emotional regulation and distress tolerance (*bodichitta*/compassion) module that is only implied in Buddhism. The reason that the emotional regulation skills are only implied in Buddhism may be due to the tendency for Westerners to require more in the way of verbal explanation. When teaching the *bodichitta*/compassion skills it is important to stress the fact that feelings *follow* in the wake of behavior and not the other way around (Appendix, Fig 5). Behavior is defined as intentional thinking, communication, and physical actions.

The four behavioral coping modules of APT differ from the Noble Eightfold Path in that they are to be learned in a non-sequential manner. This is to say, the coping behavior modules are like the petals of a flower that are connected to a central hub or core (Appendix, Fig 7). This core at the center of the four modules is none other than the Process-Self perspective. In point of fact, as with the traditional list of cognitive behavioral skills that constitute the Buddhist Four Noble Truths, the APT coping skills depend on the cultivation of realistic beliefs. In the Buddhist Noble Eightfold Path, which is also the fourth of the Four Noble Truths of Buddhism, "right views" is often listed as the first skill to master. Right views refers to both a general ability to practice reality testing through the application of reason and critical analysis; and also, the view of the self and phenomena as being empty of an eternal and unchanging nature. In the same way, the four APT modules act to support the insight into the selfless nature of reality or the Process-Self perspective. At the same time, the APT coping skills are designed to increase moral behavior, deepen awareness, and increase the ability of the patient to regulate strong emotions and to endure crisis. All of which leads to a shift in self-concept from the static Object-Self to the more adaptive and flexible Process-Self perspective.

A breakdown of the four behavioral coping skills modules of APT are:

The Discernment Skills (Prajna, Right Views)
- Check the facts. Realistic beliefs.
- Be objective
- Label (identify and describe thoughts, feelings, sensations)
- Acceptance 1. Mentally identify aspects of your life that you cannot change
- Workmanlike attitude
- Set your mind on completion
- First things first

107

- Small steps
- Easy does it (take a relaxed, easy approach to skill-building)
- Think about the other person's emotional experience
- Think about the other person's point of view
- Balance reason and emotion
- Plan ahead
- Weigh the pros and cons

The Ethical Action / Karma Skills (Right Behaviors)
- Be honest
- Be humble
- Mean what you say and do
- Congruent communication (no mixed messages)
- Determined effort/follow through
- Do what works. Effective, ethical behavior
- Be decisive
- Constructive family relations that are hopeful, constructive, fair/balanced
- Define roles and rules in positive terms
- Non exploitation. Principled occupation and work. No exploitation of people, nature, or self
- Be helpful. Community involvement

Insight Skills (Samadhi, Right Mindfulness)
- Notice thoughts, feelings, judgments, and   sensations
- Stay in the present
- Engage fully into the experience
- One thing at a time. Single focused concentration (one-pointed concentration)
- Intend to be focused (internal mental effort)
- "6 R" it to Recognize, Release, Re-engage smile, Relax, Return, Radiate
- Acceptance 2. Mindfully include all thoughts, objects, feelings, or sensations
- No black and white verdicts. Non-judgements
- Non-attachment (engage and let go)
- No mind-reading
- Go inside
- Direct Experiential Realization/Suchness (seeing beyond mental filters or labels)

- Recognition of Higher Power
- Momentary thought stopping (mouna)

The Compassion Skills (Bodichitta, Right Feelings)

- Reframing
- Sublimation (challenging emotions into constructive actions)
- Accelerated Emotional Integration (AEI) (challenging emotions into a neutral state)
- Emotional Refinement (challenging emotions into their positive state)
- Paradoxical Intentionality (PI)
- Adaptive regression by distracting with fun activities
- Humor
- Self-soothe with the five senses
- Make things better in your environment
- No drama zone
- Be optimistic about outcomes
- Have faith
- Be grateful
- Be forgiving
- Positive Self Talk (emphasis on hopeful constructive, and fair outcomes)
- Be hopeful about one's self, people, and the future
- Movement (walk, dance, exercise, etc.)
- Relaxed breathing (deep, full, connected)
- Conscious relaxation (yoga, meditation, tai chi, etc.)
- Positive self-attributions (I am lovable, I am capable, I am worthy)
- Be assertive (gently but firmly assert your position)
- Self-care
- Connect with others (be pro-social and get involved in a healthy way)
- Centering (shifting focus to your hara or one-point)
- Intentional Spontaneity/Aimlessness (alter routines within the routine)

We can come to a deeper understanding of their use and healing potential by taking a closer look at the APT behavioral coping skills.

Coping Skills Key
The Discernment / Thinking Skills
(Accurate Understanding, Wise Views)

The discernment or thinking skills are designed to help us to arrive at an accurate understanding of life. By cultivating accurate understanding we can penetrate the interdependent and interconnected nature of reality. We can also increase our ability to see the relationship between cause and effect. Problems can only exist within a chain of events leading up to, and following, the actual problem situation. By learning to take a mental step back we can gain psychological distance from otherwise emotionally charged experiences.

CHECK THE FACTS

Emotions can seem more real than thoughts. This is especially true of toxic emotions like anger, fear, and sadness. When we check the facts we challenge our emotional thinking with reason and logical investigation. In this way we start to rewire our brain to be less emotionally reactive to adversity. A good way to begin is by deconstructing the series of events leading up to the problem situation. For instance, we might ask ourselves to examine our role in creating the problem. Other factors might include the time of day, physical health, or stress. We might also investigate those actions that are reinforcing the problem. A behavioral diary is a powerful tool that is often used to analyze the chain of events, thoughts, and behaviors preceding and following a crisis. For example:

1.) **The triggering event** - oversleeping. 2.) **Thoughts** - "Oh no, I can't be late for work. This is the second time this week. The boss will fire me!" 3.) **Feelings** - anxiety, panic. 4.) **Behavior** - rushing around trying to get ready; driving too fast on the freeway.

A behavior diary can help us to break down and understand the chain of events that go into how we react to a given situation. In this way we can begin see our part in creating the situation. From this perspective we can decide on how we might utilize our coping skills to counter any negative reactions.

BE OBJECTIVE

Objective analysis of the situation asks the question, will an unbiased observer agree with my analysis? Am I being truthful with

110

myself? Does my analysis make sense? Along the same lines as checking the facts, the skill of being objective allows us to look at both sides of a situation. Because of our personal biases we tend to align with a point of view that we find comfortable. In so doing we neglect the need to evaluate the argument on its own merits. By being objective we come to a more balanced conclusion regarding any number of questions in life.

LABEL IDENTIFY AND DESCRIBE
Label, identify, and describe the feeling or sensation, e.g., pain feedback, emotions, or intuition. Before we can begin to manage our feelings we must first be able to identify them. By failing to identify our feelings we are at their mercy. Therefore, the skill of identifying and assigning a label to our feelings is essential to putting some distance between feelings and behaviors. Simply saying "I feel okay" or "I feel bad" does not provide us with the necessary insight into our emotional life. What is required is that we put a name to our feelings if we are to understand their origins. Our emotions also have a physical aspect. For this reason, we must also learn to describe how our feelings manifest in our body. "I feel tightness in my chest and my palms are sweaty. I seem to be feeling anxiety. This might be related to my upcoming trip to see my relatives this weekend." Having identified and described our feelings and sensations we can now utilize other coping skills to help us manage them.

INTELLECTUAL ACCEPTANCE
Intellectual acceptance is a mental process of thinking about those aspects of a situation that are unresolvable. If it is raining outside this is a fact and we must accept it. It does us no good to become upset about the rain or ask to ourselves if we, somehow, brought it on due to our bad karma. Intellectual acceptance is different from experiential acceptance because it utilizes reason. Using the skill of Intellectual acceptance we set about to analyze those aspects of a situation that are simply beyond our control. After doing so we are better positioned to change those aspects of the situation that we can influence.

SET YOUR MIND ON COMPLETION

Anyone who has ever run a five kilometer race knows the importance of keeping the finish line in mind. If we visualize giving up, the chances are that we will quit halfway through. Setting our mind on completion is the same as setting our intentions with regard to any other task. Most people have had the experience of setting our intention on waking up at a particular time in the morning without an alarm clock. We simply tell our deeper mind to wake us up at six a.m. The same principle applies to the skill of setting our mind on completion. Setting our intention is not the same as mentally forcing our mind to think in a certain way. When we mentally grasp at a given outcome we tend to push it away. In some cases, mentally grasping at an outcome will actually attract the opposite of what we are trying to achieve. However, if we gently allow the idea to resonate in the back of our mind we are more apt to succeed. In meditation we set our intentions on non-grasping, unconditional acceptance, and *metta* or loving kindness. We then imagine these intentions dropping like stones into a clear pool of water. Now we can enter into meditation without having to worry about maintaining our intentions. They are already working away in our deeper mind while our conscious mind settles into stillness, joy, and calm. Throughout our meditation our intentions will remind us to let go and open up to the here-and-now. But for the most part they operate out of sight.

FIRST THINGS FIRST

Decide the best time and place to begin any endeavor. Even before we can break the problem down into smaller pieces, we must figure out where to begin. Often, the very place to begin is by deciding to break the problem down into smaller parts. We might also begin by seeking advice or doing research. Another tactic is to make a list of all the things that we need to consider and them putting them into a logical sequence.

SMALL STEPS

The best way to tackle a large problem is to break it into bite size pieces. The thought of cleaning and organizing one's entire house can feel overwhelming. However, if we plan on doing one room at a time the task becomes less intimidating. The same principle applies to mastering the APT coping skills. At first the list of coping skills may seem too extensive to even contemplate. But by learning one set of skills at a time the entire task becomes fairly easy.

EASY DOES IT

Easy does it means to pace yourself and avoid burnout. Western society tends to reward productivity and hard work. The idea of taking a day off just to relax in the middle of the week seems lazy somehow. But if we use the skill of checking the facts we come to a different conclusion. People in the Western world suffer from more stress related illnesses and complaints than any other population on earth. The skill of pacing ourselves is critical to long term mental and physical health. Slow and steady wins the race.

THINK ABOUT THE OTHER'S EMOTIONAL EXPERIENCE

Think about the other person's pain without getting caught up in their suffering. Don't take ownership for their feelings or try to fix them. To Think about the other person's emotional experience is different from getting caught up in them. When we *think* about how someone else might feel we engage our intellectual rather than our emotional mind. At first glance this may seem uncaring and cold. After all, doesn't the word compassion mean to feel the pain and suffering of others? And where this may be true in the strict definition of the word, the skill of thinking about the feelings of others is more of an analysis than empathy. We must first have an intellectual understanding of another person's feelings before we can safely engage their feelings. To lead with empathy runs the risk of becoming emotionally enmeshed. Becoming enmeshed produces a codependent reaction on our part. The essence of codependency is the desire to control our discomfort by supposedly helping the person who is in distress. We don't want to feel our own agitation at the suffering of the other person. Therefore, in an effort to avoid agitation we seek to rescue them. But this attempt to save the other person is only a control maneuver. It is for this reason that we must avoid codependency by using the skill of thinking about the other person's emotional experience.

THINK ABOUT THE OTHER'S POINT OF VIEW

Along with the skill of thinking about the other person's emotional experience is the skill of thinking about their point of view. Human beings develop different sensibilities about right and wrong, good and evil, and what constitutes appropriate behavior. It is not our place dictate what others should believe. Rather, we are better served to consider how they might have come to see life in a particular way. There are many dynamics that play into the development of a person's worldview. How we were raised as a child, cultural influences, and socio-economic status all affect how we see the world. We are also influenced by our gender, age, and a host of other factors. Before we judge someone else for their beliefs we might first use the skill of thinking about the other person's point of view. In this way we can defuse many conflicts before they begin.

BALANCE LOGIC AND EMOTIONS

Integration skills (reason and feeling, knowledge and experience, etc.). Find the creative blending of thinking and feeling, i.e., "Wise Mind" (Linehan, 1993, p. 109). Buddhism teaches us to walk the middle path between extremes. Common sense suggests that we that we avoid excessiveness in most situations. However, sometimes it seems as if there is no middle path to be found. We cannot halfway murder or harm another person. Not killing is an all or nothing commitment to take the side of compassion and kindness. The answer to this seemingly insurmountable contradiction is to find the integration between two extremes. For instance, suppose we set out to purchase a new automobile. Unfortunately, when we arrive at the dealership the salesperson informs us that our only color selections are black, white, or some variation of grey. If we limit our understanding of the middle path as making a choice between black, white, or grey, we will end up with a disappointing car buying experience indeed! Fortunately, we know enough to step out of this black and white dilemma by taking the best of each value to come up with a fourth option: color. The integration of logic and emotion is wisdom or experiential understanding. Wisdom combines intellectual understanding with feelings derived from actual life experience. From the perspective of wisdom we do not judge the mistakes of others because we have been there ourselves at some point. Instead, we seek to guide and support without becoming preachy or morally superior. The skill of balancing logic and emotions, knowledge and experience, or any other extremes frees us to express our values and moral principles in a wise and compassionate manner.

PLAN AHEAD (STRATEGIC THINKING)

Being strategic is an important skill to learn in life. However, we must be careful to include the genuine welfare of others when being strategic. Being strategic means that we think through the consequences of our actions in an objective manner. "If I do A, then

B will most likely be the result. However, if B falls through I can always try plan C or plan D." Using the skill of being strategic we plan for the future but from the standpoint of the here-and-now. We are also careful to think about how our actions might affect the feelings of other people. It is poor strategy to make enemies and to burn bridges in life. Sooner or later we might reap the consequences of our thoughtlessness by way of recriminations and retaliations. Wise strategy includes the good of everyone, and in so doing, better ensuring our own highest good as well.

WEIGH the PROS and CONS:
Another skill that can help us in making better choices is to weigh the pros and cons. The first step is to make a list of reasons for doing (pro) something versus not doing it (con). Then we reverse the procedure by making a list of pros of *not* doing a thing versus cons of *not* doing a thing. In this way we can make sure to cover all the bases. For example, one of the pros for buying a house is that it is an economic investment. On the other hand, a con for buying a house is that it comes with hidden fees and upkeep expenses. A pro for NOT buying a house is the freedom from responsibility that comes with renting. A con for NOT buying a house is the loss of a sense of ownership and permanency. Whatever method we use, weighing the pros and cons is often helpful in making difficult decisions.

The Ethical Action / Behavioral Skills
According to Buddhist psychology karma is defined as cause and effect driven by choice. We cannot say that it is karma without the element of human volition. Suppose the wind loosens a pebble that then triggers an avalanche. This would be an example of simple cause and effect. Should a human being choose to cast a pebble that then triggers an avalanche, it is karma. The difference between the two lies in the act of self-determination. The good news is that karma is not imposed on us from outside. Nor is it cosmic payback for our good or bad past life deeds. Rather, we generate our own karma within our minds. If we invest in destructive patterns of thinking, feeling, and behaving we poison our mind-body system. Our relationships will suffer as well. But when our actions are established in wisdom and compassion we reap the rewards of peace, health, and prosperity. At the end of the day our wellbeing is determined by what

we do. And what we do begins in the mind and then moves outward like ripples in a pond.

BE HONEST

The skill of being honest begins with ourselves. It takes courage and faith to drop our defenses and look at our own pain. Fear, anger, sadness, and desire are natural feelings that everyone possesses. In and of themselves these feelings are just another form of emotional energy. However, because we cling to false notions of how we should be, must be, or have to be, we tend to attach a level of self-identity to our feelings. If I feel angry then I must be out of control. I *should* have more control. If I feel fear, it means I'm a coward. I *must* be fearless. If I feel sadness or desire it means I am a weak person. I *have* to be strong. By being honest with ourselves we can then relate to others from a place of sincerity. We no longer have to hide behind a façade of who we think we should be. Nor do we have to lie about our feelings and intentions. Now we can be honest with others as well. This being said, we are also mindful that some truths can hurt people. Knowledge before one is ready can do more harm than good. But rather than resort to lying to protect ourselves, we simply assert that we do not feel comfortable talking about certain subjects at this time. In this way we can be honest while acting from our values.

BE HUMBLE

Humility is the doorway to genuine self-esteem. Because we practice humility we no longer need to feel superior to others. We are free to relax and just be. Now we can open our hearts and our minds to wisdom and guidance. We are like the proverbial empty cup that has plenty of room for new things. If our cup is already full we cannot add even a single drop of new wisdom or knowledge. To learn new things, we must be humble. We must admit that we do not know everything there is to know. By practicing the skill of being humble we are able to hear the advice and suggestions of our teachers, mentors, wise friends, and family members. People sense our humility and feel safe around us. We can take risks because we do not fear making mistakes. We can be the student rather than the master. We can be ourselves.

BE KIND (GOLDEN RULE, METTA)

The cultivation of loving kindness or "*metta*" in Buddhism is a critical aspect of learning to tame the mind. On the surface, it may seem that kindness would not need to be the focus of a coping skill. However, in the absence of intentionally cultivating loving kindness we can easily fall into the habit of treating others harshly. We may come to take our gruff and angry attitude as a sign of strength or character. There is also the real danger of becoming proficient with our coping skills but lacking in empathy. In such cases we can use our ability to regulate our feelings at the expense of the welfare of others. We might act out selfishly and dismiss the harm our thoughtlessness causes as being the problem of the other person. Where it is true that we cannot directly make another person feel a particular feeling, we do have the ability to influence the feelings of others. The end result is to harm both ourselves and the people around us by inspiring resentment and animosity. It is for this reason that the cultivation of advanced coping skills must include the practice of kindness to be balanced and healthy. Loving kindness is not the same as presenting a false face of caring. Rather, it is a decision to treat others as we would ideally wish to be treated ourselves. By cultivating kindness we draw out similar feelings in everyone we interact with.

MEAN WHAT YOU SAY AND DO
The line between childhood and becoming an adult consists of taking ownership of our decisions. It is by embracing the power of taking responsibility for our actions that we begin to feel free. Before we were at the mercy of fate; but now we can say, "This is my choice and I will face whatever consequences – good or bad – that might be the result." We mean exactly what we say, and our actions reflect this. Other people can trust us to follow through and to be accountable. We earn the respect of others and we respect ourselves.

CLEAR COMMUNICATION
Clear communication means that we don't give mixed messages or demands, e.g., "Tell me how to solve my problems *but* don't give me advice!" "Isn't so-and-so a jerk? *And* how dare you attack my friend." We do not generally set out to give mixed messages. Instead, mixed messages are the result of not being clear about our intentions. We might want to vent our frustration about the actions of a friend. But at the same time we feel guilty about attacking someone we care about. If we are not mindful we can end up speaking out of two sides of our mouth. This can be especially harmful when a parent disciplines a child using mixed messages. The child hears that they

should not behave in a certain way; but, at the same time it is also a joke. The child does not know what to take away from this. Is this misbehavior or is it funny? Should I succeed or fail? Children are asking adults to tell them what they should do. By giving them mixed messages they become angry and anxious. If this pattern continues into adult life the world might seem to be a confusing place. We may become indecisive and uncertain and our communication style reflects this. By practicing the skill of congruent communication we align our actions and intentions with our values and principles. In so doing we communicate our highest good – both verbally and non-verbally – into positive outcomes for ourselves and others.

FOLLOW THROUGH

Once we determine our course of action we then go through the steps to reach our goal. Along the way we might feel like giving up due to self-doubt. However, having "set our intention" we are ready to practice the skill of following through. We can use the skills of small steps and breaking the big problem into smaller pieces if this helps. We can have a workmanlike attitude and pace ourselves to avoid burnout. We might even decide to change direction provided we have weighed the pros and cons and checked the facts. We can use the skill of paradoxical intentionality to push past our internal resistance to change. By practicing the skill of following through to the end we are building on our successes. In time we can look back on all that we have accomplished. Now we can rest assured that we can reach the goals that we have set out to achieve.

DO WHAT WORKS

Using the skill of doing what works we shift our focus to finding solutions rather than obsessing about problems. We are not in denial that problems exist. But instead of avoiding problems we reframe them as being challenges. In this way problems become stepping-stones to positive change. Now we are on the way to finding out what works in any given situation. We can focus on solutions to our challenges and take effective steps to resolve them. However, we are mindful not to violate our values and principles in the name of "finding solutions." Our solutions are powerful because they are founded upon our sense of integrity.

BE DECISIVE

Even before we can set our intentions we must decide what to set them on. In the process of coming to the point of decision we might weigh the pros and cons and check the facts. Now we can be confident that we have all the information we need to be decisive. We can gather our intentions and act in a direct and effective manner. Using the skill of being decisive we can cut through the doubt and fear that might otherwise derail us. We follow through to the end empowered by our intentions that are aligned with our actions. Everyone has had the experience of trying to decide which restaurant to go to among a group of friends. One person leans toward Chinese food and another Mexican. No one can agree or make a firm decision. Instead, everyone defers to the other and so nothing gets decided. By being decisive we either resolve the matter or someone else steps up with an even firmer decision. One way or the other a decision gets made and dinner is served.

DEFINE THE ROLES AND RULES

The value in defining the roles and rules is that everyone understands how to best relate to others within the group. When we understand our role we know what is expected of us. Furthermore, because the role is clearly defined we have the choice to step into the role or not. If this is not a good role for us, we simply decline. Problems arise when the roles are assigned by unconscious group dynamics. These are roles that are given to us in childhood and force us to act out a part that we might not wish to play. The role of the identified patient or bad seed is a common one. The unconscious group dynamic demands that someone play the role of the troubled child for the purpose of containing the family rage or guilt. In this way the dysfunction is maintained. No one has to look too closely at their own destructive patterns of thinking, feeling, and behaving. No one has to change. Along a similar line is the way in which the rules are stated. Rules are critical to maintaining healthy boundaries in a group. Positive rules tell group members what is expected of them. For example: we agree to disagree about sensitive subjects and to speak respectfully to one another. A negative rule only tells us what not to do. An example of a negative rule is: no cross talking or side conversations during the meeting! On the surface this might seem like a reasonable rule. However, it does not tell us what we should be doing. Can we still speak in a disrespectful manner so long as we

119

don't cross talk? Maybe we can make rude noises, scoff under our breath, or roll our eyes? A positive way to state this rule might be; we respect the speaker who has the floor. When the rules tell us what is expected of us the group, interactions become more harmonious and positive.

NON-EXPLOITATION

The skill of non-exploitation means that we do not use or take advantage of others. On the personal level we are sincere in our dealings with the people in our lives. We do not manipulate others for our personal gain or take advantage of their feelings. With regard to our occupation we do not engage in the selling of illegal drugs, weapons, or sexual exploitation. We are respectful of nature and consider ourselves to be stewards of our planet. We are also respectful of ourselves by taking care of our health and avoiding excess. We practice a sober lifestyle and are always seeking ways of bringing balance to mind, body, feelings, and spirit.

BE HELPFUL

It is not enough that we look after our own healthy self-interest. Because we are all interconnected in this world we must include the welfare of others along with our own. At every level human beings need each other to survive. Be it the nation, the community, or the tribe, we are all in the same boat. For this reason, it is to our advantage to get involved and help out. When we show up and lend a hand we make friends and, sometimes, important connections. We find that the win-win scenario is far more beneficial than the go-it-alone, self-centered way of looking at life. We take satisfaction in being part of a group that is making the world a better place. No contribution is too small. Be it pouring coffee at a recovery meeting or volunteering to be on a committee, we gain a healthy sense of pride in our contributions to the common good.

The Insight Skills (Wise Concentration; Mindfulness)

Co-equal to the discernment and ethical action skills is the insight/awareness skills module. One of the main objectives of this set of behavioral skills is the cultivation of non-judgmental, experiential awareness more commonly known as mindfulness. Mindfulness is like the warm illumination of a candle that radiates from a bright center. In recent years the practice of mindfulness has been promoted as a staple in both mental health and self-help circles.

However, without the discernment skill of setting one's intention, even the practice of mindfulness runs the risk of becoming a rote mental exercise. Therefore at the beginning of formal meditation the client is instructed to set their intention on non-grasping, unconditional acceptance, loving kindness (*metta*), and staying present. By setting and sustaining their intention they can continually re-energize mindfulness. Another important aspect of insight building is the practice of one-pointedness. One-pointedness is the skill of *gently* concentrating on one thing at a time. It is like the flame at the bright center of a candle that burns without any particular effort. In Buddhism one-pointedness is referred to as absorption. Absorption works alongside mindfulness to steady the mind. One-pointedness and mindfulness unite giving rise to various states of experiential understanding called *jhanas*. "The jhana states that open the door to illumination are divided into two major groups: absorption concentration and insight meditation" (Kornfield, 2008, p. 320).

NOTICE
All too often we miss out on the simple beauty of existence as we rush to attain the next desired goal. We literally forget to stop and smell the flowers, taste the fragrant cup of tea, take in the sunset, or any number of experiences presented to us by life. In our frantic efforts to control the events of the day we neglect the moment. The skill of noticing challenges us to take frequent thirty second pauses within our twenty-four hour day. In the space of thirty seconds we simply pay attention to the many textures, smells, sounds, and tactile sensations that a given moment affords us. We learn to look at the shadows of the leaves of the tree rather than at the leaves themselves. We take in the spaces between the leaves and the branches instead of its familiar shapes and colors. Out of habit we tend to reduce the tree to a cartoon cutout. We assume that we know all that there is to know about it. But when we stop to notice, with the eyes of mindfulness, we begin to see that the same old tree is really very miraculous. It is not just "our tree in the front yard" anymore. Rather, it is a life form that reflects color and texture; light, shadow, and space. It is a wonder of nature that is connected to all other things.

STAY PRESENT
Keeping our attention on the present moment can be challenging even for advanced meditators. The brain is designed to react to the

constant flood of information channeled to it via the five senses. Making matters even more complicated is the fact the brain has trillions of neuro connections. This is why it is best for beginning meditators to find a particular time of day to practice. It is better to meditate in a quiet place with little to stimulate the brain. As your concentration improves you can experiment with walking meditation. A good way to strengthen the neuro connections that are responsible for concentration is to remain mindful while performing a simple task. Doing the dishes, cutting wood, folding clothes, etc., are examples of uncomplicated tasks that can be undertaken as a mindfulness exercise. It is probably a good idea to avoid attempting to practice mindfulness meditation while driving. With time one can be mindful while doing any activity. However, for the beginner it is safer to limit one's experiments to simple and safe situations.

ENTER

Using the skill of entering fully into our current activity depends upon truly engaging the entire experience. The person with an undisciplined mind will sleepwalk through every task. They take little notice of the textures, sounds, play of light, and all the other information their senses are offering to them. Instead, they are caught up in imaginings about the future or memories from the past. Perhaps they are investing in a personal fiction in which they are the hero or the victim? Maybe they are replaying an argument they had with a coworker? The mindful person, on the other hand, is taking in the richness of their experience. They are fully involved with whatever they are doing no matter how seemingly insignificant it may be. For on a more profound level of awareness no moment of existence is without importance. This is because every action can be a doorway to a deeper sense of reality. It makes no difference whether they are taking a sip of coffee, writing a great novel, or taking out the trash. The mindful person enters completely into the activity as if it were the most important moment of their life.

ONE-POINTEDNESS

Buddhism refers to the act of doing one thing at a time one-pointedness. One-pointedness and mindfulness are like the two sides of a coin. Core awareness is the metal that joins the two sides together. Core awareness is our natural, free flowing state over which we superimpose our small sense of self or ego. Within core awareness are the enlightenment factors of wisdom and boundless compassion.

Mindfulness is a general sense of attentiveness that is established in the present moment. One-pointedness, on the other hand, is a gentle but steady sustaining of concentration on a single subject of meditation.

Outside of formal meditation practice one-pointedness is doing one activity at a time rather than multitasking. If we are brushing our teeth, then that is all we are doing. If we are lifting a heavy box, then lifting is the only thing we are concerned with doing. Our mind is not off doing ten things at once at the expense of our current activity. However, this is not the same as being obsessive-compulsive. One-pointedness is a *relaxed* focusing of the mind on a single subject or activity. It is balanced by mindfulness and opens our awareness rather than constricting it. When we practice the skill of one-pointedness we develop the mental qualities of collectedness, equanimity, and tranquility.

INTEND TO BE FOCUSED

At the beginning of meditation it is best to set our intention. We do this by directing our deeper mind to remind us to be mindful and one pointed throughout the meditation session. We can also direct our deeper mind to bring in the energy of *metta* or friendliness to our session. This is a powerful way to break down the false divisions between ourselves and the universe. To use the skill of intending to be focused we can either tell ourselves in words, visualizing an image, or both. We can tell ourselves, "Remember to be mindful and one-pointed during this meditation." Then we can visualize the directive dropping like a stone into a pool of clear water. When intending *metta* we can start by imagining ourselves and then extending the energy of friendliness to our own mental image. We then picture a spiritual friend (not a family member) with whom we have a platonic relationship. We extend *metta* to that friend. Lastly, we let the image dissolve into formless energy. We then imagine the energy of *metta* radiating from our brow or heart center. When our attention drifts we can reset our intention as many times as needed.

"6 R" it to Recognize, Release, Relax, Re-engage smile, Return, Repeat as Needed

The 6 R method of reducing stress and struggle in meditation is a mental script that can be practiced almost anywhere. Meditation teacher Doug Kraft describes the series of Rs as a way to remember the steps of Buddhist mindfulness meditation. The first R in the series is to recognize or see the distraction that has taken us out of mindfulness. We then release our hold of the distraction using the skill of non-attachment (recognize and release). The next two Rs in the series are to relax or soften and re-engage the smile. Once we relax or soften the tension we must fill the remaining void with a positive feeling. The simplest way to do that is to smile. If we do not fill the void, there is the possibility that our old negative mental scripts will rush in (relax/soften and smile). Next we return to the subject of our meditation in order to reestablish mindfulness and one-pointedness. This can be our breathing or some other mental object that serves as an anchor to the present moment. Finally, we remember to allow the energy of *metta* (loving kindness; friendliness) to radiate like the bright light of a beautiful candle flame (return and radiate). With repetition the 6 R method becomes automatic so that we can run through the script without much effort. (Note: it is not necessary to use the 6 Rs unless our attention has drifted completely from the here-and-now).

EXPERIENTIAL ACCEPTANCE

Experiential acceptance is about being willing to open up to even our most painful feelings and sensations. We are not trying to do anything about our thoughts, feelings, sensations, and perceptions. Rather, we are simply giving them room to be. On the other hand, intellectual acceptance involves thinking about those things in life that we are powerless to change. Using the skill of experiential acceptance we practice including unalterable things without trying to change them (unless we are able to). For instance, suppose you have a headache and have already taken an aspirin. Beyond this point all that remains for you to do is to open up to the pain feedback signal. At the level of experiential acceptance pain becomes a mere sensation. It is neither good nor bad. Instead, it registers as information that is intended to warn us that something is off in our mind-body system. By developing the skill of experiential acceptance we are learning to "accept the things that we cannot change" at a deeper and more powerful level (Sifton, p. 277, 2005).

NON-CONDEMNATION

Investing in value judgments and condemnation is like carrying around a bag of heavy rocks. We are loaded down by the needless weight of our judgments and end up hurting ourselves. But when we drop our judgments we feel a tremendous sense of relief. We no longer have the burden of deciding what is right and wrong for other people. We can let other people take their own moral inventory as we attend to ours. We are off the hook and can now look after our own principled behavior. Furthermore, we can abandon our defeatist verdicts about our self-worth. By practicing the skill of non-condemnation we come to understand that the so-called "enemy" is just like us in many ways. They too are only human and are dealing with delusional thinking and suffering. They too are the product of their family system and society. And like us they seek to connect and to be happy. Judgments limit our ability to see people in their entirety. By dropping our judgments, we can expand our capacity to see ourselves and other people with clarity and compassion.

NON-ATTACHMENT
When we turn our attention inward we see that our thoughts, feelings, and sensations are continually coming and going. If we watch long enough we can begin to see patterns of thinking and feeling that endlessly repeat themselves. These patterns of thinking and feeling are made of images, memories, and beliefs that combine to generate our internal reality. By utilizing the skill of non-attachment we begin to create some psychological distance between our subjective self (the observer) and our thought patterns. Not all thought patterns are harmful. Patterns that produce feelings of kindness and compassion are to be encouraged. Likewise, those patterns that increase our ability to make wise and reasoned decisions are considered to be favorable. It is only those patterns that produce suffering and grasping that we must learn to non-attach from. Meditation teaches us to catch and release, negative patterns. We notice our patterns and accept them without judgment, clinging, or pushing them away. We then soften any mental tension associated with the patterns and let them go. The skill of non-attachment is central to neutralizing the destructive effects of craving and addiction.

NO MIND-READING
All too often in life we imagine that we know what other people are thinking. We may become uncomfortable in public if we make a mistake such as lose our footing or drop something. Immediately we assume that people are snickering at us or judging us. It is under such circumstances that we can use the skill of no mind-reading. For in truth, if we were to ask these supposedly judgmental people to

confirm our suspicions we might be surprised. It is more likely that they would express concern for our wellbeing rather than make sport of us. It is even more likely that they did not even notice our faux pas. Most of the time people are concerned with what they themselves are doing, did, or plan to be doing. We are our own favorite subject, as it were, and so have little room left in our mind to think about the actions of other people. It is only when those people are close to us and require our attention that we think about them. The likelihood of a total stranger investing time and energy in thinking about us is slim at best. When we feel that we know what other people are thinking we should take a moment to remember the skill of no mind-reading.

GO INSIDE

There is a part of our mind that is already still and at peace. It is sometimes referred to as "pure awareness" or the watching aspect of the mind. "Pure awareness is a good alternative term [for self-as-context] because that's all that it is: awareness of our own awareness" (Harris, 2009, 173). Using the skill of going inside we can watch the comings and goings of our thoughts, feelings, and sensations from a detached perspective. The subject (us) observes the object (thinking, feeling, sensations) without getting caught up in them. Pure awareness is not the same as core awareness. In pure awareness there is still a subtle sense of separation or duality. Core awareness, on the other hand, is just awareness. It has neither a subjective watcher, nor an object of which to be aware. Going inside to see the world from the perspective of pure awareness is critical for learning non-attachment. It is by mastering the skill of non-attachment that we learn to let go of suffering born of grasping. But first we must be willing to go inside and see.

DIRECT EXPERIENTIAL REALIZATION

Direct Experiential Realization (DER) is arrived at by looking deeply at a given phenomenon from the perspective of mindfulness. An example of a given phenomenon might be that of a drinking cup. For the cup to exist it depends on the empty space within the cup. Without the empty space the cup cannot exist as a container for liquids. It would be nothing more than a solid mass of ceramic. Furthermore, the cup also depends on the space surrounding the cup to exist as an object. We should also consider all of the people and steps that went into the formation of the cup. Someone had to refine the clay to make the material for the cup. Someone else had to design the cup. Still another person had to glaze and fire the cup. On and on the cup traveled from raw earth to its place in our cupboard. The very word "cup" is a mental label that is superimposed over the cup-phenomenon. Using the skill of DER we can reach beyond the label to have an intuitive experience of the absolute nature of the cup. Seen from this perspective it is more than an inert object in which to pour our coffee. Rather, its essence is that free flowing vibration and change in-the-moment. And with each passing moment the cup is created and recreated; born and reborn. Using DER we can intuitively perceive the multidimensional and interconnected nature of the cup. It is this direct experience beyond all labels that is referred to as suchness or "signlessness" in Buddhist psychology. "The greatest relief is when we break through the barriers of sign, and touch the world of signlessness; nirvana" (Hanh, 1998, p. 149). If a given phenomenon can be experienced as signless then all phenomena can be understood in the same way – including ourselves. It is the free flowing nature or signlessness that best describes the true nature of reality. From this perspective of signlessness it is possible for suffering to be transformed into the energy of wisdom, compassion, equanimity, and joy.

RECOGNITION OF HIGHER POWER
Recognizing our higher power is a process of discovery rather than invention. If you have ever picked up a friend at a busy airport, then you can understand the difference. At first all you can see are a crowd of strangers. You have faith that your friend is somewhere in the crowd, but you have yet to spot them. Suddenly the crowd parts and there she is. She was there all along. But because of the distractions and mass of humanity you could not see her. Perhaps she was right in front of you as she walked toward you across the terminal. Nonetheless, her face blended in with all the others until you had a moment of recognition. Now you can see that she was there all along. So it is with our higher power. As to the nature of what we intuit our higher power to be, that is up to us. Be it God, Christ, Buddha Nature, Allah, or some guiding principle of life. . . the important thing is that we cultivate a moment-to-moment connection with it.

MOMENTARY THOUGHT STOPPING
The skill of Momentary Thought Stopping is aimed at putting our mental brakes on our racing thoughts. In meditation this is called the practice of *mouna*. Momentary thought stopping can be achieved by

taking three, slow mindful breaths and counting up to the number three. At the end of each exhalation silently count one, two, or three and then start over again as needed. In time it will only be necessary to count one set of three for your thoughts to quiet down. Once your thoughts and their associated feelings are calm it is easier to utilize other coping skills. For instance, if you are upset and your mind is racing you can use momentary thought stopping as a way to segue into the Six Rs. In this sense momentary thought stopping is like first shifting into a neutral gear so that you can then shift into a positive gear.

The Compassion, Kindness, and Emotion Skills
(Heart-Mind)

The fourth domain of the four behavioral coping skills modules consists of the compassion, kindness, and emotion skills. Although Buddhist psychology speaks in terms of feelings, which are more generalized than emotions and moods, it is often helpful for Westerners to talk about mastering specific emotional regulation behaviors. *Metta* or kindness is the desire for all beings to be happy. Compassion is the desire for all living beings to be free from suffering. A good place to start with regard to emotional regulation is by being kind and compassionate to ourselves.

REFRAME

Reframing is when we change how we think about a situation to change how we feel. If we "frame" or think about a situation in such a way that we see only the negatives, we will tend to feel worse about it. On the other hand, if we frame a situation to see only the positives we end up in denial. The best way to frame a situation is to do so in a realistic way. We can ask ourselves, is the situation really that bad? Is there nothing left in our life that we can be grateful about? Destructive mental habits would have us thinking thoughts like, "I can't believe this is happening to me! Surely no one else has to deal with this kind of crap?" But if we change how we view adversity we can feel less upset during a time of crisis. The skill of reframing is aimed at being good at feeling (during a crisis) rather than expecting to feel good all of the time.

SUBLIMATION

Sublimation is the act of consciously utilizing our negative emotions for constructive purposes. Examples include working off stress at the gym, cleaning the house if we feel anxious, and doing yard work to burn off anger. Sublimation is different from displacement. Displacement is an unconscious process of redirecting our negative feelings at a safe target. It may not be safe to direct anger at our employer. Instead, we come home and kick the dog. However, when we use the skill of sublimation we are mindful of negative emotions while finding healthy ways to channel them.

EMOTIONAL INTEGRATION
Emotional integration is an advanced coping skill involving mindfulness and acceptance. A useful way to think of emotional integration is the analogy of the fire pit. A fire pit is made up of a ring of rocks and ash that prevent the fire from spreading beyond the limits of the burn area. In this analogy the rocks and ash are the mindfulness skills of non-attachment and unconditional acceptance. The fire represents our emotions. We can try to control the fire by jumping on it to stamp it out. However, by doing so we are more likely to spread sparks everywhere and so cause even more fires. We might even catch on fire ourselves. The other alternative is to surround the emotion with the energy of mindfulness. In doing so we allow the emotion to subside all by itself. We might also visualize the emotion as a wave that rises, abides for a moment, and then melts back into the ocean of our mind. Using the skill of emotional integration we simply observe our feelings without trying to deny, suppress, or vent them.

EMOTIONAL REFINEMENT
Emotional refinement takes emotional integration one step farther by identifying and using the positive aspects of negative feelings. Emotional refinement is one of the most advanced, and therefore challenging, of the coping skills. It is important that the practitioner not use it to avoid facing unresolved conflicts that may be the source of their suffering. This is why it is best to first learn it within the context of the therapeutic setting. However, once mastered, emotional refinement offers a powerful method of turning painful emotions into useful energy. Using the emotion of anger as an example, we become aware of the qualities of determination and protectiveness latent within the anger. This is to say, we reframe the anger as having a helpful function. As the wave of anger subsides we allow the positive emotional qualities to resonate within our being. We now recognize the essential emotional energy to be one of

determination to reach an otherwise blocked goal. All emotions are rooted in three basic impulses to connect with others, express ourselves, and to protect our own well-being (connect, express, protect). By practicing the skill of Emotional refinement we find the "diamond in the rough" with regard to feelings that we might otherwise view as bad, threatening, or shameful.

PARADOXICAL INTENTIONALITY

Paradoxical intentionality is doing the opposite of what we feel like doing in order to do the right thing. There are many mornings when just getting out of bed is a good time to utilize this skill. Diet, exercise, or attending a class or group after a long day at work can be challenging. The potential list of examples is very extensive. The value of paradoxical intentionality is that we learn to act against emotional ambivalence that is holding us back. Paradoxical intentionality is like jumping into a cold swimming pool on a hot day. We know that the initial shock of the cold water will give way to the refreshing feeling of relief. However, the minute or two of freezing gives us pause. It is then that we can use paradoxical intentionality to "just do it" by moving through our ambivalence. In the end we find that our fear of pain was worse than we imagined. We are stronger for having faced it and we can take a healthy pride in our ability to do what is right.

ADAPTIVE REGRESSION (Have fun)

We don't always think of making time for fun as an important way to cope. All too often fun is an afterthought or something we do in an unconscious way. When we have fun in an unconscious way we sometimes regress into a childish mindset. But when we choose to allow ourselves to have fun in a healthy way it becomes a coping mechanism. Having fun in this sense is an adaptive form of regression. Using adaptive regression, we find healthy ways to play that do not involve intoxicants, overeating, or hours of mindless television. We balance play with rest and productivity to allow for the many sides of our human nature. Above all, we find that we can let our hair down and still maintain our healthy way of life.

HUMOR

Human beings have a highly developed ability to see the funny side of life. This is not to say that there are no other animals on this planet that have a sense of humor. Like many social animals, the great apes also share in this ability. But it is only Man that has such an advanced capacity to see the absurd. Humor often acts as a safety valve when we find ourselves taking our plight too seriously. Consider the bad camping trip. This is the camping excursion where everything that could go wrong did go wrong. Now compare this camping experience to the one in which there were no misadventures. Which one made for the funniest stories to share afterwards? There are some situations for which it would be inappropriate to make fun. We must also be careful not to make fun in a way that is hurtful of the feelings of others. Humor can be misused as a form of denial by minimizing, when in fact, the situation is to be taken seriously. Nonetheless, when used in a respectful and adaptive way, humor can ease the tension in otherwise stressful situations.

SELF SOOTH
In any given moment we have five senses that we can use to experience the beauty of existence. When we do so in a mindful way we enhance our experience greatly. The skill of self-soothing through the five senses is a powerful way to reconnect with our spirit. If we find that we are becoming stressed and upset, we can take a walk around the block or to a park. We can take in the sights and sounds that nature offers us free of charge. Or we can set up a space in our home or office that is filled with objects of beauty. We can fill this space with art, incense, music, or essential oils. There are many ways that we can use the five senses to feel better when we do not feel good. Like any other coping skill, self-soothing through the five senses takes intentionality and practice.

MAKE THINGS BETTER
Whether we clean up a corner of our home or make a prayer or meditation shrine in the garden, there is always some small area of the environment that we can improve. By making something in the environment better we feel better as well. It is not always necessary to take on something big. Even organizing a corner of the garage or cleaning out a junk drawer will start the ball rolling. From a small improvement we might then become inspired to do even more. The important thing is to make our environment a reflection of our inner state of being. By attending to our living space we are, at the same time, taking care of our inner space as well.

NO DRAMA ZONE

Practice creating a psychological safe zone that extends two feet in all directions. Other people's drama is not your problem. Imagine this no drama zone as a two-foot bubble of calm that extends all around you. While other people are caught up in anxiety, frustration, or anger, you remain peaceful within your no drama zone. It is up to you to decide the condition of your emotional climate inside the no drama zone. Even if someone else is trying to draw you into their Drama-Victim Triangle, you have the power and right to refuse. By remaining in your no drama zone you can become like the calm center of the storm.

BE OPTIMISTIC

The skill of being optimistic involves challenging our negative assumptions about life. More often than not our efforts have proved successful in spite of the occasional setback. Being optimistic is very much in line with checking the facts. We can feel optimistic by looking at the cause and effect of our past successes. The fact is, when we think things through and persevere to the end we generally meet our goals. Our fears and doubts might seem to be more compelling in the moment. However, our achievement record stands on its own merit. We have been successful in many ways and therefore can be again. Building on our history of accomplishments is the foundation of optimism.

FAITH

It is said that the path to inner peace is like a difficult ascent to reach the summit of a high mountain. The way is strewn with rocks and narrow passages. However, upon reaching the summit the air is clean and the view is much better. At any point we might be tempted to give in to doubt and despair. "I can't do this; it's too hard. I should have known better than to try!" But it is in such moments of doubt that we must summon our faith. For in point of fact, doubt is nothing more than having faith in the negative outcome. Therefore we must reach deep inside to find the hidden resources of inner strength that are buried within. To do this we must choose to invest in faith. Even a single moment of genuine faith can move mountains of suffering. In time these brief moments of faith expand and deepen. As this happens we develop embodied faith that becomes part of who we are.

BE GRATEFUL

The skill of being grateful is one of the most powerful and direct methods of emotional management at our disposal. If we stop to reflect we can find many things to be grateful for. If nothing else, we can be grateful that things are not worse than they already are. This is not to deny that we have real challenges to manage. On any given day we must address problems both big and small. Rather, the skill of being grateful balances out our list of challenges. The fact that we are alive to count our blessings is a good place to start. When we practice the skill of gratitude we immediately begin to feel better.

BE FORGIVING

Forgiveness is a process of trust building. When trust is broken it is impossible to truly forgive. We can embrace the idea of forgiveness, but we cannot truly feel it. To forgive we must be willing to let go of the hurt that was inflicted upon us. But to let go we must have confidence that the offender will not hurt us again. A good place to begin the process of trust building is by establishing trust in our selves. If we can forgive ourselves for being imperfect, we can take a workmanlike attitude about our mistakes. We can reframe them as learning experiences that point us in the direction of success. Now we can begin to trust our ability to make better decisions. Having established trust, it is easier to allow genuine feelings of forgiveness into our heart. By forgiving ourselves we can now extend forgiveness to others. They too are human beings who are driven by patterns of negativity and suffering. The skill of forgiveness is one of the most challenging and rewarding of the coping behaviors. It is not easy to master, but a little forgiveness can work miracles of healing for ourselves and those around us.

POSITIVE SELF-TALK

The way we talk to ourselves effects our emotions in a significant way. If we give ourselves negative messages all day long our mood will suffer. Self-defeating statements undermine our ability to apply our coping skills. Imagine if we were to go through the day listening to a recording of someone telling us that we are stupid, ugly and unlovable? Now add to this that we are hopeless failures who are destined to screw up our every endeavor. "How come other people have it so good? Why am I such a hopeless loser? I hate myself!" Such messages can only trigger feelings of anger, anxiety, and depression. Yet, as obvious as it may sound, people fall into the trap of negative self-talk all the time. The skill of positive self-talk begins by being mindful of our self-defeating thinking. From a place of awareness we then challenge negative self-talk with accurate understanding by checking the facts. Is it really true that we never succeed at anything? What about love and respect? No one has ever loved us or shown us respect? There are over seven billion people on this planet. Can we claim to have met every one of them? How do we know that none of the seven billion people on the earth could not love or respect us? Checking our negative self-talk and countering it with realistic and affirming language, we replace destructive mental habits that lead to suffering.

BE HOPEFUL

There is no such thing as a depressed person who is – at the same time – hopeful. Hopelessness about one's self-worth, the future, and the world makes up the trifecta of depression. The skill of being hopeful directly challenges our depressed thinking patterns by checking the facts. Are we truly without value as a human being? Do we not possess the innate impulses to connect to others and to protect our own existence? For that matter, can we claim to know the future? How do we know that our fate is destined to end in disaster? Regarding the world, there are billions of people on this planet whom we have yet to meet. Can we be certain that some of them won't become our friends and allies? The hopeful perspective is founded upon a firm foundation of truth. Choosing to find things to be hopeful about will always alter our feelings for the better.

MOVEMENT

One of the best ways to improve our mood is to move. Sitting too long is harmful to the body. It is not surprising that there is an epidemic of depression in the Western nations given the prevalence of the couch potato lifestyle. People who make a daily habit of hiking, biking, or simply going for a twenty-minute walk tend to feel better than those who don't. This is why doctors prescribe movement to patients who have recently undergone surgery. It is generally recommended that people get thirty minutes of cardio exercise three to four times per week. This helps to maintain a healthy weight and to prevent anxiety and depression. A twenty-minute walk in the sunlight promotes vitamin D production. Vitamin D is essential to mood regulation and a deficiency will cause depression and irritability. The skill of movement is not to be taken for granted.

When we feel achy, upset, restless or sluggish, it is a good time to get up and move.

BREATH

Breathing is something we do all the time. In every meditative practice it is the breath that is central to establishing mental stability and calm. The breath can be used to anchor us in the moment by using it to integrate body and mind. When our breathing is slow and circular it changes the biochemistry of the brain and nervous system. Conversely, we can use faster, connected breathing to energize the body and mind. One-pointed, mindful awareness begins with being able to follow the passage of air going in and out of the lungs. It is best to let our attention settle on one area of the body rather than chasing our breath up and down the spine. In this way we avoid exciting unnecessary thought production while meditating. The skill of circular, connected breathing provides us with a quick and effective method of regulating our emotions.

CONSCIOUS RELAXATION

The skill of conscious relaxation is about softening our internal, mental tension. Mental tension results from grasping and resistance. When we grasp at a given outcome we simultaneously resist the undesirable outcome. So grasping and resistance are two sides of the same coin. Mental and physical tension arises from the interaction of grasping and resistance. However, even before we can release our mental tension we must first become aware of it. Mindfulness is of great importance in this regard. Through mindfulness we can become aware of our tension and then curious. What is it that I am grasping at? What am I pushing away? Where do I experience the tension in my mind-body complex? From mindful curiosity we can then begin to systematically soften the tension using any number of progressive relaxation techniques.

POSITIVE AFFIRMATIONS

Positive affirmations are realistic affirmations. They are affirmations that are based on the truth rather than wishful thinking. We are lovable because we love ourselves. We are lovable because there are so many people in the world that could love us. We are lovable because there is always someone in our life that has loved us or does love us. We are capable because there are many things that we can do for ourselves. The fact that we got out of bed and fed and dressed ourselves is an example. We have learned and mastered many complex tasks in our lives that we may now take for granted. We can read and write. We can drive a car or perform a job. And we are worthy because we are human. All human beings deserve to be treated with respect and kindness. If we exclude even one person, then we are opening the way for all people to be shut out. But because we all have basic goodness, Buddha Nature, or the Divine Spark, we are all deserving of respect, compassion, and kindness.

GENTLY ASSERT

Although asserting ourselves is a form of effective communication, it is central to our emotional life as well. There is always a feeling quality to how we communicate our needs and wants. Many of us have had the disquieting experience of talking to someone whose lips are smiling but whose eyes are cold. Their words seem reasonable, but their eyes tell a different story. We can sense the ill intent behind their words. Conversely, we may have also encountered someone whose words convey a serious message but from a place of compassion or concern. This might have been a counselor, doctor, or emergency worker. Asserting ourselves in a positive way is different from demanding, on the one hand, or placating on the other. When we practice the skill of gently asserting we state our intentions in a definitive way while respecting the feelings of others.

SELF-CARE

Emotional self-care depends on physical self-care as well. Too often we neglect our physical health as we push ourselves to achieve success at all costs. This results in physical imbalance leading to emotional burnout. For our emotional health to be sound we need to maintain a routine of proper diet, exercise, sleep, hygiene, and attending to injury and sickness. Regular medical and dental checkups are a must rather than an afterthought. In addition, some type of meditation that includes conscious relaxation is highly beneficial. Yoga, Tai Chi, Aikido, or some other form of moving meditation will support our health on a subtle energetic level.

BE PRO-SOCIAL

Being pro-social means to get involved with a healthy group activity or to volunteer somewhere. If nothing else go out in public at least once a day. It is not unusual to isolate when we are sick, injured, or upset. There are times when we need to withdraw in order to heal.

Nonetheless, it is important to our general well-being to maintain our social connections. This is because people are social beings by design. We do not thrive in isolation. Too much time alone results in depression, anxiety, and loss of touch with reality. Without feedback from other people we can become lost in our worries about the past or the future. Likewise, social media is not a true substitute for actual human interaction. It can, at times, serve a useful function in lieu of actual social interaction. However, it is the direct interaction between people that fulfills our need to relate. There are times when it may not be practical to meet up with a friend or family member. In such cases it can be beneficial to attend a free support group, religious service, or simply sit in a crowded café. As long as the people we are involved with are committed to a healthy lifestyle, connecting with a group is always helpful.

CENTERING

The skill of centering is aimed at becoming emotionally grounded by focusing on our sense of physicality. Our physical center is located two inches below our navel in the middle of the body. In Japanese martial arts the physical center is called the hara. The Chinese call it the tantien. In yoga it is referred to as the sacral chakra (*swadhisthana*). This is the center of free flowing emotions and physical intuition. Traditionally its color is orange and its seed sound is VAM (v-ah-m). By connecting our movements with the hara they become vastly more powerful and integrated. However, we do not need a black belt to connect with the hara. All that is required is to use our breath to shift our attention to the hara. Take a long and slow breath and mentally connect it to your hara. As you exhale imagine the energy of your hara expanding to fill up a three-foot bubble of light all around you. Nothing bad can enter this bubble. All negative energy simply bounces off of this bubble of light. At the same time feel your center of gravity becoming heavier and grounded to the Earth. Affirm to yourself, "I am safe. I am capable. I believe (in my higher power)." There are many ways to get centered and it is up to us to explore and experiment. The main thing is to find a way to reconnect with our physical sense of being in the moment. When we feel stressed and overwhelmed we can reconnect with the hara to quickly become grounded once again.

INTENTIONAL SPONTANEITY

Intentional spontaneity is a way to break out of our fixed patterns of behavior. The ego's will-to-control is the enemy of ease and grace. The central activity of meditation is to learn to let go of control while opening, unconditionally, to the here-and-now. On the one hand we need a certain degree of routine and discipline to make progress towards our goals. On the other hand, it is wise to learn to relax in our efforts to succeed. A good way to balance letting go with maintaining discipline is to vary the routine within the overall routine. An example of intentional spontaneity is to switch up our workout when we go to the gym. We can alternate the machines we use along with the order in which we use them. Another example of intentional spontaneity is to make the effort to visit places that we have not yet experienced. For instance, there may be many public parks and trails at our disposal that we have not yet bothered to explore. By practicing the skill of intentional spontaneity we allow for ease, creative adaptation, and novelty within the structure of discipline and healthy routines.

The daily use of the APT diary card is critical to the patient's mastery of APT. As with any cognitive behavioral homework assignment, the use of homework assignments such as diary cards has long become a staple with regard to the cognitive behavioral schools of therapy. "Homework is an integral, not optional, part of cognitive therapy. In essence, the therapist seeks to extend the opportunities for cognitive and behavioral change throughout the patient's week" (Beck, 1995, p. 247). Making the shift from the Object-Self to the Process-Self perspective may be challenging to the client's identity. Repressed feelings and memories are likely to arise as the client does the hard work of restructuring their core self-schema. The need to learn and utilize a variety of emotional coping skills becomes all the more important during this phase of treatment. Therefore, successful therapy depends upon the client making consistent use of the APT behavioral skills. Ultimately, the client must thoroughly integrate the APT coping skills to the point of becoming automatic. Once integration of the coping skills is achieved, the focus of therapy can move in the direction of learning life enhancing maneuvers. The difference between coping skills and life enhancing maneuvers is that the client is no longer in a state of crisis. Rather, they have learned to manage and regulate their feelings to a high degree. Now they are free to engage in learning specific processes designed to build on their success in the skill-building phase of therapy. This being said, it is important to emphasize the need to proceed at a pace that is comfortable for the client. Mastering new behaviors will always put us in direct conflict with our own deep-seated, unconscious habits.

The pace at which the client integrates the APT coping skills will vary depending on any number of factors. These factors include the client's psychiatric diagnosis, cultural background, socio-economic status, and family system. Differences in gender, level of maturity, ethnicity, and intellectual capacity must also be taken into consideration. The following is an example taken from my efforts to utilize the APT diary cards with Native-American men in a substance abuse recovery setting.

For several weeks I had been using the diary cards to help the men to rebuild emotional coping skills eroded by chronic drug and alcohol abuse. I had seen progress as the men gave examples of how they were using the APT diary cards in the process of their recovery. A breakthrough came for one of the men whom I will call "James" after a particularly challenging APT skill-building group. James had asked me for help on a written assignment that we were engaged in during the group. The assignment consisted of answering three questions related to how the group members might have felt and responded when faced with an opportunity to practice one of three central skills: Acceptance, Non-Attachment, or Accurate Analysis. James, an intense thirty-something young man, flagged me over as the group was busy working on the handout. In a hushed voice he explained that he was having trouble finding a specific skill to help him gain emotional distance from the memory of his brother's suicide. At this point I should have seen this disclosure as a red flag and been careful not to assume that James was willing to share this painful experience with the rest of the group. However, I was caught up in the task of managing ten very different personalities while trying to engage each of the men in a meaningful way. This being the case, I failed to ask James if this was something he was comfortable sharing in a group format. When his turn came to share what he had written, James volunteered to share with the rest of the group about his brother's death. However, after the group James asked to talk to me in private. As we walked around the grounds James struggled to maintain his emotions. He told me that he felt I had not been mindful of his emotional state and that he had no intention of sharing this painful memory with the rest of the men. Seeing that he was right, I expressed my sincerest regret and assured him that I would be more careful in the future. But James continued to share about the circumstances surrounding his younger brother's suicide until it became clear that he needed to work through it. Furthermore, this event in his early life had set the stage for his later descent into drug and alcohol abuse. So painful was this memory that he had been unwilling to discuss it with anyone. Nonetheless, after a month of participating in emotional skill building, James now had the coping tools that had allowed him to begin to manage his feelings of grief, anger, and guilt. By the time we finished our conversation, James admitted that he had played a part in creating this situation by not being clear with me that he did not intend to share in the group. I encouraged James to follow up with his counselor about his unresolved feelings of being responsible for his brother's suicide. We then discussed specific coping skills that would support James in his grief work. Had it not been for his willingness to learn and integrate the APT coping skills he might not have had the confidence to confront his pain. Now he would be able to let off the emotional charge of the past a little at a time armed with a greater ability to endure his most challenging feelings. Nonetheless, it was at this moment that I understood how challenging the diary cards could be. In the coming weeks I would slow down the pace of the groups by focusing on one specific skill at a time. I would continue to refer to the APT diary cards, but only as an index of coping skills for the men to refer to as they completed written exercises in the group setting.

Over time I reformatted the diary cards to be more holistic in nature which I felt to be more in line with the Native worldview. After a group session in which I had asked the men to place various traditional Native practices into one of four domains representing the four directions of the Medicine Wheel, I found that the men could not comply with my instructions. The Native Medicine Wheel is a model of a balanced worldview that also can represent the four general aspects of a human being. The four directions are commonly divided into the four races of man, Red (also Brown), Black, White, and Yellow; the four points of the compass, North, South, East, and West; and the four personal aspects of mind, body, emotions, and spirit. The men were quick to point out that Native practices fit into each of the four domains but for different reasons. A good example of the holistic nature of a Native coping behavior is the practice of traditional Native drumming. The practice of drumming includes mindfully singing prayers (spirit), learning and mastering the song and the drumming pattern (mind), experiencing a feeling in response to the drumming and singing (emotion), and the physical act of drumming (body). To try and artificially compartmentalize Native drumming into a specific domain runs counter to the unified perspective that is central to the Native worldview. In future group sessions I would ask the men to assign a given coping skill to each of the four domains of the Medicine Wheel. Having done so, they would list the different ways the coping skill related to a particular domain of the Medicine Wheel. This change in approach to learning behavioral coping skill allowed the men to better practice the APT coping behaviors with greater intentionality. Furthermore, they were able to do so simultaneously across all four domains of feeling, thinking, body, and spirit.

The APT diary cards are only a tool to be used or modified as needed for the benefit of the patient. Ultimately, the diary cards should be phased out as the patient continues to practice and embody the various APT coping skills. To this end an exit plan is included as a central feature of the end stage of therapy. In keeping with the goal of empowerment, the therapist should always strive to follow the lead of the patient. Lastly, no matter how the APT skill building component is delivered, the safety of the patient must always be in the forefront of the therapist's mind. As with any therapeutic modality, the challenge is to be responsive to the patient's instinct for healing while remaining faithful to the treatment model.

Chapter Nine
Individual Therapy

"Any reasonable approach to psychotherapy not hiding itself behind a professional jargon must be comprehensible to the intelligent layman" — Fritz Perls

The Layperson's Perspective

There is a phrase in Buddhism that refers to the direct, intuitive experience of reality: this phrase is "the emptiness beyond emptiness" (Holiday, p. 134, 2013). Reality, according to Buddhism, is empty of any static or irreducible position. This is to say, all of existence has the underlying nature of being interdependent and interrelated. Furthermore, all things exist in a state of multidimensionality or "interbeing". "In the light of interbeing, we see the flower in the garbage and the garbage in the flower" (Hanh, p. 244, 2006). From the standpoint of interbeing, we see that an ocean wave is dependent upon the ocean for its existence. At the same time, it is impossible to have an ocean without waves. Conversely, the wave cannot be said to encompass the entire ocean in itself. Ultimately, we understand that both the wave and the ocean share the underlying nature of water. The interbeing of wave, ocean, and water is that these are coexisting dimensions of the same, ultimate reality. The underlying truth of reality is that no one thing can exist separate from other causes and conditions. If we look closely with deep mindfulness we can see this is also true of our own self-nature. Nowhere in the mind or body can we find a fixed or distinct self-entity that we can separate from the totality of our being. Buddhism calls this fluid and interdependent nature of things *sunyata* or emptiness. However, unless we have a direct experience of emptiness our intellectual understanding of reality will do us little good. The subject of emptiness may provide us with an amusing topic of philosophical conversation at a coffee shop. Nonetheless, such an insubstantial insight offers only a shadow of true understanding. In this case our understanding will do little to relieve our personal suffering. Knowing this, we must take care not to stop short at a superficial grasp of emptiness. Only through mindfulness meditation and the cultivation of a deep understanding of reality can we arrive at the emptiness beyond emptiness. This is the experience of reality beyond our intellectual filters and concepts.

To be sure, there are times in our life in which we seemingly stumble, as if by accident, upon a sense of expansiveness. Psychologist Abraham Maslow referred to these instances as the peak experience. Such moments are characterized by a feeling of having surpassed the limits of our ordinary mind. We may feel a sense of being united with a force or power far greater than ourselves. In the religious realm this is often considered a time when one is touched by the divine. Feelings of love and bliss seem to illuminate the mind and body. There is a sense of being guided and protected by a great intelligence that is at once personal and impersonal. Buddhism would consider this experience to be a glimpse of our true nature. In the Japanese Zen Buddhist tradition such a moment is called a satori. Should this moment of awakening be expanded into a stable state it is referred to as a *jhana*. A *jhana* is a level of experiential, meditative understanding that is rooted in *samadhi*. *Samadhi* is defined as being in a state of relaxed but steady concentration. It is arrived at, primarily, through the practice of mindfulness meditation. Although difficult to define, the state of *samadhi* allows the yogi to loosen her grip on her attachment to the self. Having done so, she is able to experience her free flowing nature of interbeing that is imbued with innate wisdom and compassion. Needless to say, the state of satori cannot be forced. In fact, any attempt to grasp at satori will only result in pushing it away. It is better to think of the satori as a momentary awakening. Our eyes open for an instant and we see things as they really are. But then they close again leaving us with our old view of a dualistic universe. However, something of the experience remains and alters us on an unconscious level. Over and over this process continues until the day that our eyes remain open. It is at this point that we cast off delusion and become enlightened.

Let us consider another way in which we might arrive at satori. If we define satori as a momentary recognition of our core awareness, perhaps we can also identify other moments of recognition. For myself I find a glimmer of recognition by shifting my attention to the spaces between objects in my environment. Rather than focus on the cars in a parking lot, I expand my field of vision to include the spaces between the cars. I take in the light reflecting in the sheen of the car's paint. I look with the eyes of mindfulness at the leaves swirling in a dust devil. I notice textures both rough and smooth. Gradually I gain an intuition of the underlying unity and emptiness within the mundane.

I have also found that spending time in nature can produce this same effect. Whether mindfully taking in a sweeping vista, or observing the ripples on a stream of mountain runoff, I often experience a profound connection to my deeper mind. Without a doubt I am not unique in this experience. Artists, philosophers, writers, and poets have described such moments of profound insight while immersed in the wonders of nature. It is no coincidence that many of the great teachers throughout the ages have referred to natural images and examples to illustrate profound ideas and teachings.

Still another method of gaining a moment of recognition is through movement. Hath yoga, tai chi, and aikido are powerful forms of moving meditation. If performed in the right spirit they have the potential to assist the student to connect to the infinite. I like to think of this point of connection to be a place in the limitless continuum of being. It is like a band on a spectrum that begins in the place where we are standing and extends to the universe. By learning to reach past our personal fictions – the stories that we make up in our minds and in which we are the central character – we can have a direct, intuitive experience of the entire continuum of being. And in doing so, we can learn to let go of worry, doubt, and desire that obscures our recognition of our core awareness.

Our human nature is the home of our Buddha Nature. This is the place in our deeper mind that is already awake and serene. The term, Buddha Nature, has a dual meaning: it refers to the possibility that anyone can awaken to their true nature of free flowing peace and love. It is also synonymous with ultimate reality. In answer to the Zen kaon, does a dog have Buddha Nature? The answer is that, from the standpoint of ultimate reality, a dog *is* Buddha Nature. Therefore, the best place to discover our Buddha Nature (core awareness) is within our everyday human nature. In my work with clients I use a number of psychotherapeutic maneuvers designed to lead the client to have recognition of their core awareness. The process involves examining one's current situation just as it is. Once the client has taken a step back from their attachment to their personal fiction they can be guided to the recognition of their core awareness. I call this method the reprocessing maneuver or RM. The client is guided through a standard round of cognitive behavioral processing that has problem identification as its primary goal. The underlying working model or schema is brought into conscious awareness where it can be analyzed. The meaning and the feelings associated with the schema are discussed in the context of the client's past. However, it is at this juncture that the RM changes direction. Rather than assign homework designed to challenge and restructure the schema, the client is led through a process of detachment to non-attachment. The end result is to allow the client to discover – by way of an intuitive recognition – the rich resources latent within their own core awareness. Once having become aware of their wealth of inner assets the client is better equipped to do the work of restructuring their dysfunctional working models.

Another method of helping a client to have recognition of their core awareness is by listening to the account of their lives for moments of awakening. These are instances in which the client has unconsciously crossed into a state of process. The process state is characterized by having an experience of the self as being fluid and adaptive. When a person is in process they have ceased to grasp at the notion of themselves as being separate from their environment. Emotions are integrated or are instantly transformed into a positive manifestation. The mind is not caught up in personal fictions or in interacting with super ego objects. There is a sense of being at one with an underlying intelligence that is part of a unified whole. Our perception of time vanishes or speeds up so as to seem almost non-existent. Within the context of therapy, the client may not be aware that they have made a shift in perspective from their personal fiction and into core awareness. They only remember that, at this moment of their lives, tasks that seemed otherwise beyond them have now become effortless. They may have arrived at their Process-Self by facing their fears or surpassing their own expectations in some significant manner. Perhaps they came upon a natural vista that moved them in a profound way. It is at this moment that the client has unintentionally entered into a state of deeper, more expansive, awareness. However, lacking the language to define or understand this shift into the Process-Self perspective, the client might come to believe that some external agency was behind their experience. As a therapist I strive to make the client aware that such moments are quite natural, but often overlooked, aspects of the human experience. I refer to such instances as a person having a moment of recognition of their Process-Self. Once the client has had a moment of recognition pointed out to them, I encourage them to pay attention to similar moments of recognition. In time the client learns to be increasingly mindful of recognition moments. Now they can use these occurrences as a way to shift into process at will. In this way the client will discover that inner peace is not something outside of themselves that must be hunted down. Rather, they will come to understand that free flowing ease is our natural, underlying condition. What is required on our part is the willingness to practice with skillfulness, ease, and courage. It is in this way that we can come to a lasting recognition of our core awareness, imbued as it is with infinite intelligence and boundless compassion.

From a therapeutic standpoint the question is, what is it that is standing in the way of a client's experience of recognition? To answer this question we need to examine their underlying attachments to false beliefs or fetters. Buddhist psychology identifies ten major fetters to inner peace that give rise to the five hindrances or negative mind states.

The ten fetters are:

The belief in a separate self-entity that exists behind the eyes. In some cultures, that sense of self is felt to exist in the hara and in others in the heart center.

The belief in the negative outcome. This is also the fetter of doubt.

The belief in the power of ritual and magic.

The belief that sensual pursuits will lead to happiness and inner peace.

The belief that anger is an effective means for controlling people and circumstances.

The belief that achieving an idealized life circumstance such as winning a lottery will lead to happiness.

The belief that going to a formless, heavenly realm will lead to happiness.

The belief that one is spiritually superior to others.

The belief that one's core sense of self can be annihilated.

The belief that material objects have a separate self-nature.

Therefore, a central concern of individual therapy is to identify and challenge the client's underlying fetters to awakening. In doing so their delusional state of mind will diminish and their ability to express their core awareness will increase. This will allow them to shift into a state of unfettered continuous process. From the standpoint of process, they increase their ability to experience all of their thoughts and feelings without judgment or shame. This is to say, they can respond skillfully rather than react.

We do not have to be afraid of our feelings once we learn to relate to them in a skillful way. When we stop trying to close off to our experience of our emotions we begin to relax. We can allow for the full range of emotions without judging ourselves for being human. We find that we can express our feelings in a constructive manner rather than venting or suppressing them. However, before we can arrive at such a level of emotional efficacy we must examine the patterns of negativity that hinder our ability to manage our feelings.

The Clinical Perspective

The executive director of a resource family agency once asked me what my personal mission in life is. I responded without hesitation, "To extinguish suffering one moment at a time." Later I would add the goal of empowering people to inner peace. It is to these ends that APT is directed, one way or another. APT therapy sessions, whether for an individual or a group, should always include these overarching goals. No matter what the presenting problem, the clinician must be able to include the goal of empowering the client to live a happy life. Equally important to the goal of happiness is the goal of helping the client to extinguish their personal suffering. Failing this the therapist is not doing APT and should switch to a therapy that will better accommodate the patient's concerns. Furthermore, the clinician must do so in language that is best suited to the patient's worldview.

With regard to individual APT, it is best that individual therapy take place in unison with group Auto Process Therapy. One reason for this is that fostering self-esteem through building mastery of the four APT competency modules increases significantly with group reinforcement and feedback. "Self-esteem and public esteem are highly interdependent. Self-esteem refers to an individual's evaluation of what he or she is really worth, and is indissolubly linked to that person's experiences in prior social relationships" (Yolam, 1995, p. 57). Consequently, it is fair to assert that the clinician is not truly practicing APT in the absence of linking individual therapy to group practice.

Another significant consideration pursuant to the importance of linking individual and group therapy is the element of narcissistic self-absorption. "Many patients enter therapy with the disquieting thought that they are unique in their wretchedness, that they alone have certain frightening or unacceptable problems, thoughts, impulses, and fantasies" (Yalom, 1995, P. 5). Without a doubt, individual therapy runs the risk of reinforcing the patient's sense of being unique in their personal experience of suffering. However, by including group therapy as an important component of healing, the patient can better come to realize that they are not alone in their distress. It is this understanding of the universal nature of human suffering that elevates us beyond self-pity and opens the way for increased compassion (*bodhichitta*). Indeed, the most profound understanding of compassion, in the Buddhist sense, springs from attaining a deep understanding of the interdependent nature of reality. "When we look deeply into the nature of interdependence and see that the person harming us is also a victim – of his family, his society, and his environment, understanding arises naturally" (Hanh, 2006, p. 204). It was this deep understanding into the universal human condition that motivated the Buddha on his quest for enlightenment and the extinction of suffering. "The Buddhas and Patriarchs, because of their great mercy, have left open the vast gates of compassion in order that all living beings, both human and celestial, may thereby realize enlightenment" (Soto Shu Sutras, 1982 p. 30).

Lastly, even the most seemingly benign skill-building oriented group therapy can have the unintended effect of re-traumatizing patients. "Groups can act as powerful catalysts for personal change, and they can also pose definite risks for group members" (Corey, 2004, p. 62). The exposure to other patients' painful histories during group can trigger PTSD and unresolved family of origin issues. For this reason, it is both prudent and sound to pair any form of group process and psychoeducation with an individual therapy component.

As with most forms of psychotherapy, the application of individual APT begins with a comprehensive assessment of the client in context of the larger system they inhabit. It is the *client-in-context* standpoint that marks a shift from the idiosyncratic Object-Self to a Process-Self perspective. "Clinical social workers view clients and their problems in relation to the multiple contexts in which problems occur" (Sands, 1991, p. 2). To best accomplish a systems perspective of the patient-in-context, a biopsychosocial clinical assessment that includes both the APT theoretical perspective and the clinical model is recommended. Such an assessment is one that includes both symptomology and a theoretical perspective. Following the completion of the biopsychosocial assessment, the treatment plan, setting of goals, objectives, and interventions is developed.

Beyond standard office management, safety and crisis practices, and general referrals, APT looks at the beginning stage of therapy as a stabilizing time. To better achieve stabilization of the client the use of the APT diary cards, both in the individual and group therapy setting, is employed early in treatment. Even for the patient with a highly cohesive ego function, making the shift from Object to Process-Self can be challenging to the patient's self-concept and ability to regulate their feelings. Providing the patient with stabilizing emotional fallback strategies and group support can reduce unnecessary anxiety related to the restructuring of the self-schema. "Self-evaluations and self-instructions appear to be derived from deeper structures: namely, the self-concepts or self-schemas" (Beck and Freedman, 1990, p. 36).

Allowing for resistance to change, another important component of the opening stage of therapy is the therapeutic agreement or client contract. It is not unusual for a patient to push against the very interventions that might help them to move towards their treatment goals. "Resistance responses are normal during counseling" (Miller, Rollnick, 2002, p. 99). Therefore, in order to better respond to and anticipate the normal resistance arising between therapist and patient, it is helpful to co-create a client agreement in collaboration with the patient. Such a client agreement would include, in the very least, the following elements:

- A no-harm clause: do not harm self or others.
- Daily use of the APT diary card.
- Weekly attendance in APT group therapy.
- Completion of any homework.
- An agreed-upon contingency plan for noncompliance with treatment assignments.

Having assisted in drawing up the terms of the treatment contract, the client is more likely to comply with the agreement. The rationale for involving the client in formulating the terms of the therapeutic agreement is that it is the patient who is the ultimate expert on his or her own self-growth. "Given a free choice, and in the absence of external force, individuals prefer to be healthy rather than sick, to be independent rather than dependent, and in general to further the optimal development of the total organism" (Corsini, Wedding, p. 140, 1995).

During the middle (working) phase of therapy the emphasis is on helping the patient to achieve their personal goals of therapy within the greater context of APT. This means that both the patient and the therapist must keep in mind the central goals of APT. To reiterate, the overarching goals of APT are to extinguish suffering and to make the shift to the Process-Self perspective. Central to realizing these goals is the cultivation of non-attachment, also non-grasping. Grasping takes the form of specific attachments to false beliefs that fetter us to the Object-Self perspective.

The fetters number ten in all and operate mainly in the unconscious mind. As stated in Chapter Three, the fetters are: belief in a permanent and independent self (Object-Self); doubt in the Noble Eightfold Path or treatment; and the belief in the efficacy of ritualized magical thinking or religious practices (superstition). The next fetters on the list are the belief that sensual pleasure is an end in itself (addiction); the belief that power leads to happiness (aggression); and the belief that one is spiritually superior to other people (narcissism). The sixth and seventh fetters are the belief that attaining an idealized self-identity living under better circumstances will lead to lasting happiness. This is the fetter of materialism. Following the attachment to the belief in an idealized material existence is the attachment to being reborn into an idyllic formless realm. Rather than fully engage their life on earth, this fetter would have the client longing to die and ascend to the Christian Heaven, the Buddhist Pure Land, or some such other divine realm. Both of these fetters are manifestations of infantile regression. The remaining fetters are the fear of existential annihilation (anxiety) and the belief that external phenomena have an intrinsic self-nature (narcissistic object infusion). Understanding the exact nature of the client's fetters is an important aspect in devising a course of treatment. It is to this end – the cultivation of non-grasping to false beliefs as a treatment goal – that the use of the APT reprocessing maneuver (RM) can be employed.

There are two ways in which to utilize the RM. The first application of the RM is as a specific therapeutic maneuver. The second way to apply the RM is as a general format to use in structuring the entire session. In the former, the therapist guides the patient through the four stages of the RM during the course of a single session. In the latter, as a general way to structure a session, the entire session is divided into stages one through four without direct reference to the RM. This is to say, the principles of the reprocessing maneuver are utilized without employing the formal reprocessing maneuver itself. In this case, the therapist keeps in mind the goals and format of phase one of the RM: (1) Construct a problem statement out of the patient's problem story that they bring to the session, and (2) Identify the underlying thought distortion, e.g., "I am unlovable," "I am helpless," "I am worthless." Verbalize it in the patient's own words. (3) Externalize the thought distortion by stating it in terms of being a person *with* a thought about being unlovable, helpless, or worthless. At this point the therapist might discuss methods that the patient can use to gain psychological distance from their thoughts and feelings without actually guiding the patient through the stages of detachment to non-attachment. Because it is not the therapist's intention to lead the patient through the RM maneuver per se, the therapist is free to approach the session from any number of directions.

In the next part of the session the therapist would hold the meta-perspective of phase two of the RM. In phase two the task is to help the client to process their thoughts, along with any feelings associated with the thoughts. During phase one and phase two of the RM the course of the session has followed a standard cognitive approach. In this phase the goal is to uncover and raise (by increasing emotionality within the safety of the therapeutic setting) the patient's conscious awareness of their maladaptive thought distortions. Only by increasing emotionality can unconscious thought distortions surface. Following the process of raising thought distortions is the work of challenging them. It is this tactic that forms the basis of most traditional cognitive-behavioral schools of therapy. And in fact, it would be at this point that the therapist and client would design homework to be practiced between sessions, and together in vivo. But in APT, with its goals of psychological reorientation of the self and the cultivation of non-attachment, the session would continue into phase three and four of the Reprocessing Maneuver.

In stage three of the RM the patient is instructed to visualize themselves floating above the challenging situation like a bird hovering in the sky. The situation, along with all that is taking place in the mind, is seen from the perspective of detachment. The patient is then asked to articulate what they think about the situation, their thoughts about the situation, and finally their feelings about the situation. However, when conceptualizing the entire session in terms of the RM, the therapist would only *suggest* that the patient see the situation from a "bird's eye view". It must be noted that this is not the same as using guided meditation as in the RM to give the patient an experience of being above their mind. Rather, it is only a metaphor for looking at one's challenges from a more objective standpoint. In either case, when teaching a patient any form of mindfulness meditation it is important to make them aware that a delayed reaction is not uncommon. Such a delayed reaction often comes in the form of repressed memories, thoughts, and feelings breaking through into conscious awareness. It is for this reason that the patient must be firmly grounded in the APT coping skills. It is equally important that the therapist be available to the client in between sessions and to provide the patient with emergency contacts. Finally, the patient is led through the detachment to non-attachment mental exercises (see Chapter Seven) by way of practicing making the segue from the Object to the Process-Self perspective. It is at this point in the session that the use of formal mindfulness meditation can be employed.

Mindfulness meditation is generally taught by instructing a student or client to simply sit while observing the inhalation and exhalation of their breaths. I recommend limiting one's attention to the passage of air in and out of the first quarter inch of the nostrils. This prevents the mind from chasing the breath up and down the spine and so inadvertently increasing the production of automatic thoughts. In some cases the client will feel more comfortable focusing on the air as it enters and leaves their lungs or abdomen. This will work just as well provided the client's attention remain on a specific region of the body and not shift continually from nostril to lungs to abdomen. The goal here is to let thought production settle down in a natural manner. I often instruct a client to keep their eyes open and gazing softy at a single point in front of them. However, it is also acceptable for the client to keep their eyes closed if they prefer.

When the client's concentration wanders, as it eventually must, the client is instructed to smile and return to the focus of their meditation. The gentle returning to the focus of concentration is what, in Buddhism, is referred to as one-pointedness. Throughout the meditation session I remind the client to utilize the "Six R" method of maintaining the qualities of kindness and non-grasping. "Bhante emphasized ease. When the mind's attention was pulled away, I was to first just recognize where my mind had gone. Then I was to release or let go of the distraction, relax, smile, and return to the primary object of meditation. He called this the Six Rs" (Kraft, 2013, p. 19). It is important that the client sit upright, either with their feet flat on the ground or, if the client prefer, seated cross-legged on the floor. In either case, their back should be straight. If the client is sitting on a chair then have them move slightly forward to about midway in the seat. They should not be reclining their back against the chair or a wall, but rather sitting upright and independent. This encourages awareness and helps to prevent falling asleep. If they are sitting on the ground then any position they can be comfortable in will do. In such instances sitting on a flat cushion or in a half lotus position is recommended. Beyond these basic instructions I then tell the client to not fight against or judge their thoughts, feelings, or sensations. Rather, I encourage the client to allow their cognitions and feelings to simply come and go. The client must be instructed to let go of grasping at control. In place of control, mindfulness meditation uses a relaxed and easy approach in focusing one's concentration. It is this state of mind, in which the flow of feelings, thoughts, and sensations arise and fall away naturally, that is the mind of non-attachment. Following these general mindfulness guidelines, I prompt the client to describe what they were most aware of in terms of body, feelings, thoughts, or mental objects. I ask the client to reflect on what they think went well with the session and what they might have done differently. This is not a judgment on their performance but a way of prompting the client to look more closely at the process-nature of their own mind. I may then follow up by asking the patient to consider the main thing they got out of the meditation session. Lastly, I will ask them how they might apply what they took from the meditation session in their everyday life.

Throughout the individual therapy session the therapist will be looking for opportunities to prompt the patient into a state of *recognition* of the Process-Self perspective. As the therapist listens to the patient's story the therapist will point out those instances in the patient's narrative in which the patient was in their Process-Self. An example of recognition presented itself when a client described learning to scuba dive. In spite of having gone through hours of the prerequisite classes and training, when it came time to dive into the ocean the client panicked. She became overwhelmed with feelings of dread and began thrashing around in the water. At this point her diving instructor stopped her and told her to simply let go and fall into the water rather than attempt to control her body. To her surprise, when she let go and fell forward she was able to swim quite naturally. After she recounted this event to me I pointed out that she had demonstrated a shift in perception from her Object-Self to the Process-Self. This is to say, she transitioned from the perspective of being a *self* that was attempting to control her body, to that of a *process-being* who was already at one with her body and her environment. Using her experience of scuba diving as an example I was able to prompt the client to identify other moments of recognition.

Teaching a patient to recognize those moments when they have shifted into a Process-Self perspective can be challenging. This is because the shift in perspective is often subtle and easily missed if one does not know what to look for. For this reason it can be helpful to illustrate for the patient what the Process-Self versus Object-Self looks like. One such illustration is that of a hypothetical situation in which a woman is going through her morning routine. From the Object-Self perspective her mind is fuzzy, and her actions are on autopilot, even as the alarm clock goes off to announce the new day. The automatic thought arises in her mind, "It's too early! I can't handle this!" The thought of it being too early generates an emotional response of resentment and sadness. Without any real connection to her physical body or to the present moment she makes her way to the bathroom. Her mind plays out a script of what the morning should be like while her body follows through her ordinary routine by the force of habit. She notices a pain in her lower back and silently curses as she pulls away from the feedback her body is giving her. She drinks a cup of coffee but never really tastes a drop of it. Instead, she is caught up in daydreams of how much happier she was when she was in her twenties and going to college. Her ten-year old daughter walks into the room and says, "Hi Mom." The woman murmurs a reply without looking up from her coffee. And so the day continues with the woman sleepwalking her way from one task to the next. She lives vividly in her mind while only semi-awake to the actual experience of reality in and around her. As she performs a host of activities she is caught up in an internal narrative of "I" "Me" "Mine" that defines her sense of self. She ends her day as she began it . . . tired, sad, and resentful.

I then ask the client to imagine the woman having the same experiences, but from the Process-Self perspective. The alarm sounds the beginning of a new day. She takes a moment to scan her body and focus her consciousness even before sitting up and putting her feet on the floor. She is aware of the habitual thought that "It's too early" and the rise of resentment that follows it. However, she counters the thought by embracing it with mindful acceptance. She then proceeds to set her intention on doing the opposite of what she feels like doing. In one breath she mindfully sits up and sets her feet squarely on the ground. She lets her thoughts settle down for a moment as she follows her breath entering and leaving her nostrils. She neither clings to, nor pushes away her thoughts, feelings, and sensations. Rather, she expands into them while allowing them to pass away one after the other. All is included. All is let go. Letting go of grasping, she becomes one with the moment.

Even before she enjoys a cup of morning coffee she takes the time to do a few stretching and breathing exercises. Now she is fully grounded in the present moment and ready to engage, mindfully, any challenge the day may offer. She feels the cool morning breeze through the patio window and she remembers to be grateful for the steaming cup of coffee, for her health, for her many blessings. But more than anything she is grateful for her family. She smiles as her ten-year old daughter comes into the room. "Come here, baby," she says as she gathers her daughter up in a hug. And so the day continues.

A central goal of APT counseling is to help the client access and free her own internal resources. Standing in the way of this goal are the client's unconscious attachments or fetters. Therefore, in order for her to realize her own hidden strengths, the client must address her unconscious fetters. To this end the APT therapist will employ a variety of therapeutic maneuvers, including the Cross Dialectic, The Reprocess Maneuver, regular review of the APT behavioral coping diary cards, and teaching the safe use of the advanced emotional regulation, integration, and refinement maneuvers. In any given session the focus of therapy can shift between skill-building on the one hand, to aiding the client to have a recognition of the Process-Self perspective on the other. In other sessions the goal of therapy is the deep restructuring of the self-schema leading to a profound shift into Process-Self. Regardless of the APT maneuvers the therapist chooses to utilize, the overarching goals of APT remain the same; to help the client to extinguish personal suffering while empowering them to connect with their intrinsic nature of inner peace.

Chapter Ten
A General Overview of APT Group Therapy

"In interactional psychotherapy, also, process has a specific technical meaning: it refers to the nature of the relationship between interacting individuals" — Irvin Yalom

The Layperson's Perspective

Buddhism teaches that liberation from suffering must include the welfare of all people if it is to be fully realized by the individual. This is because love and compassion serve to bridge the emotional gap between people in a way that the intellect, by itself, cannot. Thinking about the other person's emotional experience is a good beginning. But it takes empathy to complete the connection between self and others. In the absence of empathy we run the risk of falling prey to feelings of self-pity and resentment. Stewing in isolation we might imagine that we are unique in our suffering. We may feel as if no one else in the world has ever gone through such trials as we have been subjected to. It is in these moments that the shared group experience can help to shake us out of our narcissistic reverie. Taking refuge in the spiritual community (*sangha*), recovery group, or psychotherapeutic support group is often our best defense against depression, anxiety, or substance abuse born of isolation. It is for this reason that APT was designed to be delivered in both an individual and group therapy format to be most effective.

A compelling group dynamic is generated as clients form bonds of trust through talking about their individual challenges and triumphs. The group dynamic is frequently taken in surprising directions by the force of the group members' sharing with regard to healing. The topic of the group may begin with reviewing the APT skill-building diary cards but then open to a discussion about the skill of direct experience of reality (DER). This is often the case when practicing therapeutic group meditation and reflection. It is the interaction of the group members that makes this possible. The individual therapy setting is limited to the interaction between the client and the therapist. This is useful for deep insight building but it does not necessarily serve to reinforce the client's sense of connectedness.

With regard to the group dynamic and the APT diary cards, the power of the sharing aspect of the support group cannot be overstated. Within the group format a client can explain how he was able to use the various coping skills that he utilized throughout the week. In this way the other group members may gain insights into new ways in which to employ the APT coping skills they might have not yet considered. Using the example of being stuck at a traffic light, a group member might list the skills of acceptance, emotional integration, and reframing to help with anger and frustration: "I was waiting at the red light behind another car and I noticed a bumper sticker on the other car that read: Mystery Spot – Santa Cruz, California. Right away my mind went to a trip I took to Santa Cruz last year. I found myself wanting to be on the beach and NOT stuck in my stupid car waiting for the light to finally change! I could feel myself knotting up inside and getting angry. But then I remembered to use the skills of temporary thought stopping and taking three mindful breaths. After that I was able to reframe my thinking about the situation. I mean, at least I have a car that runs. . . and it's paid for. I also used acceptance by thinking that I can't control traffic and I don't have to be out driving if I don't really want to. But what I *can* influence is how I respond to being in traffic. So, at this point I imagined my anger as being a wave and I let it sink back into my mind. It took a few minutes; but by the time the anger wave was gone the light had turned green."

The shared group process can be used to advance the skills required for learning mindfulness meditation. After reminding the group members of the basic meditation instructions and the rationale for meditating (to practice mindful non-grasping) the group is instructed to "sit in mindful acceptance" for a given number of minutes. Once the allotted time has passed the group facilitator will end the meditation and allow each group member to share. In this way the group members can provide important feedback to the group facilitator. The facilitator can then offer ways to fine tune the meditation with the goal of teaching the skills of non-grasping (also non-attachment) and experiential acceptance. For example:

Group facilitator: "How did your meditation go? What were you most mindful of this time?"

Group member: "For me it was peaceful. I noticed a lot of birds and traffic sounds. Also, I could see a squirrel that was running around by the trees over there. It reminded me of when I was a kid and we would go camping. But then I remembered to 'Six R' it and I came back to the present."

Group facilitator: "That's great! So you didn't grasp at being in-the-moment?"

Group member: "I started to; but then I remembered to be relaxed about it. After that I got really quiet and peaceful."

Group members often begin to combine the APT coping skills in creative ways as they become more familiar with them. It is not uncommon to use one of the discernment skills such as "checking the facts" before attempting to use an advanced coping skill such as emotional refinement: "I was feeling like people were staring at me when I was at the grocery store the other morning. But then I remembered not to 'mind-read' and to 'check the facts.' I looked around at the people in the store and I noticed that they were totally focused on what they were shopping for. I doubted if any one of them could pick me out of a lineup for a million bucks! So I took a moment to let my anxiety melt back into my mind; but I tried to keep the positive part of the anxiety. Sure enough, after a few seconds a great feeling of humor popped up and I almost laughed out loud right there in the store. Imagine if I had! Then people really *would* be staring at me."

When group and individual therapy are combined they reinforce each other in powerful ways. APT behavioral skill-building – which is the primary focus of group therapy – allows the client to go deeper into their personal insights. Insight building – the focus of individual therapy – is enhanced by the skill-building aspects of group therapy. Together they work to provide a firm foundation for change and growth.

The Clinical Perspective

Group therapy is sometimes viewed as a matter of adjunct therapy that is often brought up as a consideration in the closing stage of therapy. It is not uncommon for patients to be referred to a therapy group after they have worked through the middle stage of treatment. To be clear, one cannot be said to be practicing APT in the absence of a group therapy component at the very outset of treatment. The reason for this is that APT depends on the Buddhist concept of the sangha, or community, to be effective. "The Sangha acts, in the main, as a support group that helps each member to reinforce the often challenging skill building aspect of Buddhist training" (Noss, 1999, p. 168). And as with most support groups, the free exchange of each member's triumphs and struggles in a non-judgmental setting offers insights and encouragement to the group as a whole.

By the same token, APT group therapy is severely limited if practiced in the absence of individual APT therapy. More and more mental health agencies are funneling patients into various theme-based groups that lack an individual therapy component. The rationale is that individual therapy is expensive and time intensive compared to the group therapy format. But if we are to remain true to the APT treatment model a patient must have both the group and the individual APT therapeutic experience. Without this concurrent dual exposure the patient may not benefit fully from the combined skill-building and the insight building aspects of APT.

There are a number of ways in which to structure a group, such as process versus focus group or structured versus open; but no matter the overt form the group takes, in APT, having a consistent underlying structure ensures the core principles of the group are reinforced in each session. To approach the APT group format in the absence of a core principles orientation is to run the risk of the group degrading into a techniques driven group therapy approach. "Techniques are quite useful tools both as catalysts for group action and as devices to keep the group moving. But techniques are just tools, and like all tools they can be used properly or misused" (Cory, 2004, p. 455). Such an underlying structure, in the case of APT, is founded upon referencing the four coping behavioral modules and the central theme of Process-Self reorientation. By referencing the content areas in each group, the overall group structure can be open-ended, while at the same time ensuring fidelity to the treatment model.

In terms of APT group therapy design, it is up to the therapist to decide how to tailor a group to a given population of patients. For instance, an APT group for people in substance abuse recovery will have different goals than a group for patients with mood disorders or relational issues. Likewise, patients struggling with PTSD will differ in terms of group goals from personality disordered patients. In addition, the element of cultural diversity must be included in both individual and group therapy for therapy to be effective. Nonetheless, consistent throughout all APT groups is the emphasis on skill building and unhooking from the Object-Self while identifying with the free flowing Process-Self of the moment.

Many of the more common elements of group therapy can be researched in the general psychotherapeutic literature already in circulation. Consequently, it is not my intention to reiterate the basics of group therapy. For example, as a therapist I like to include the use of a Tibetan prayer bell to call patients to mindfulness and/or to point out judgments and attacks in a non-critical way. The use of such a device is hardly original but is often effective, as are many other common group therapy practices in general circulation. But underlying all group therapy is the importance of breaking out of isolation by openly verbalizing one's private experience of suffering and triumph to others who share similar struggles. The aforementioned process of verbalizing one's private experience to the other group members is defined by Yalom as "universality" (1995, p.5). The feedback the patient experiences, as well as the validation from the other group members is often more therapeutic than the content areas of the group. For it is often in the process of group dynamics *between* patients that insight and healing takes place.

In every relationship interpersonal interactions serve as a mirror in which we can discover previously hidden aspects of ourselves. "Generally, one's sense of self is formed by observations of oneself and of other's reactions to one's actions" (Linehan, 1993, p.4). Often it is not the other person in the relationship that serves as the mirror. Rather, it is the relational interactions between people that serve a self-reflective function. In terms of group dynamics, the potential for relationship based self-reflection is magnified by several factors including personality differences, individual complaints, and group member personal sensibilities about life. For this reason, it is the role of the group facilitator to ensure that the mirror of self-reflection remains undistorted by bias, judgments, and projections. It sometimes happens that the potential for accurate reflection fails when emotions run high and the group dynamic runs too far afield. Therefore, as in individual therapy, it is of paramount importance that the therapist be ever mindful of transference and counter-transference.

APT group therapy is aimed towards the development of both intra-personal and inter-personal coping behaviors. For this reason, the APT group therapy format is uniquely suited for couples or family therapy. Since effective communication is essential to healthy interpersonal relations, it is entirely possible for the clinician to design any number of APT group therapy formats – including APT family and couples group therapy. In point of fact, one may argue that effective communication, along with the ability to regulate one's own thoughts and emotions, increases the overall harmonious interaction of couples and within the family system. "Consider that 80% of communication between people is non-verbal, [and] speaks directly to the feedback loops which occur between two people" (Forbes, Post, 2009, p. 23).

Lastly, it is not the objective of this book to design a pre-formatted outline for an APT group therapy; instead, it falls upon the clinician to be creative and to innovate with regard to group design and content. As long as the focus is on promoting the four APT competencies modules and unhooking from the Object-Self, the APT group can take any number of forms. In this manner, the momentum generated between group members and the facilitators can inform the group as a whole in dynamic and unexpected ways.

Part Three
Addendum
Beyond Process Self

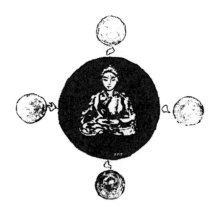

Chapter Eleven
Towards a Therapeutic Path to Enlightenment

"The Truth is simple but the Way of Man is hard.
First you must learn to control your Self" — Robert A. Heinlein

A note to clinicians: according to Buddhism, the possibility of the complete and lasting cessation of human suffering is an attainable possibility. Such a state of being is characterized by abiding inner peace, kindness, compassion, and direct insight into the process nature of reality. It is this state of being that is called enlightenment in Buddhism. In the following chapter I have outlined what I consider to be the beginning of a therapeutic path to enlightenment. This is not meant to be a concise roadmap by any means; rather, I am attempting to begin a discussion about the potential utility of Western psychotherapeutic methods towards this end.

All of my life I have been drawn to sweeping vistas, winding paths, and open spaces. In such moments I have gained an intuitive recognition of ultimate reality. . . what some would call God, Source, or a higher power. And where many people reach out to their higher power with words, rituals, or prayers, I prefer to connect with ultimate reality in silence. For any label I attach to it only creates the mind of separateness. In his book, The Awakened Mind, Geshe Tashi Tserling writes, "Peel away all the layers of delusion that currently cloud our minds and what remains is a pure, unfettered mind of love and complete understanding, our Buddha Nature." If I must call my intuitive recognition of ultimate reality by a name, I will call it the deeper mind. As for ultimate reality itself, it cannot adequately be put into words. Rather, it can only be recognized with the wisdom eye – *ajna* – that directly perceives the true nature of all things.

The word *enlightenment* holds many connotations for different people. Even among Buddhists, enlightenment is difficult to pin down with precise definitions. The Buddha was said to remain silent when asked directly to define the state of enlightenment. Instead, he would point the student back to their own process of self-realization. The Buddhist teacher might ask the student, "Who is the one who is asking the question?" The question, of course, is a device or *koan* designed to force the student to go beyond the limitations of the ordinary mind. The end result is to have an awakening (*satori*) to the deeper mind, or Buddha Nature. The reasons for this reluctance on the part of Buddhist teachers to talk about enlightenment may have to do with the risk of inadvertently inflating the ego. If enlightenment can be reduced to an intellectual description, then any intelligent person can claim to be enlightened. Furthermore, the state of enlightenment depends upon a direct perception of reality beyond our cognitive filters. Still another reason may be that the experience of enlightenment is a uniquely personal one that cannot be over-generalized. Nonetheless, there are some Buddhist scholars who have attempted to provide us with a clearer understanding of enlightenment. Such teachers include Thich Nhat Hanh, Bhante Henepola Gunaratana, and Geshe Tashi Tserling.

In volume three of his six volume series of Buddhist psychology books, The Foundation of Buddhist Thought, Geshe Tserling defines enlightenment as a state of mind having the mental factors of calm abiding, compassion, loving kindness, and "direct yogic perception" of ultimate reality (2006, p. 131). The mental factor of calm abiding consists of being able to suspend discursive thinking combined with vivid intensity of perception. Compassion refers to not wanting others to suffer – even those who have harmed us. Loving kindness is the desire for others to find happiness. Direct yogic perception of reality refers to the experiential understanding of emptiness or *sunyata*. Emptiness is understood by Buddhists to mean the selfless, process nature of both phenomena and person. When all of these mental factors are present, then a temporary state of liberation from suffering is said to have been attained. However, this is not the same as supreme or ultimate enlightenment. With regard to ultimate enlightenment, there is a final cessation of suffering predicated upon rooting out delusion on every level of consciousness. Needless to say, such an accomplishment is rare and can only come about after many years of dedicated work and training – several lifetimes according to many Buddhist teachers. "Liberation [from suffering] can be achieved within lifetimes, it is said, enlightenment takes three countless great eons" (Tserling, 2006, p. 134).

From a therapeutic standpoint the temporary cessation of suffering and the subsequent empowerment to inner peace is possible for anyone, to some degree. Only individual circumstances and limitations determine to what degree the client will be able to meet these fundamental goals of APT. To better understand the mental factors that combine to create a temporary state of enlightenment I will break each of them down into discrete elements, or mental factors, of consciousness.

- **Calm Abiding:** a mental state arrived at through the practice of a brief suspending of attachment to discursive thinking along with enhanced attention to the present moment (vivid intensity). Geshi Tserling refers to the temporary suspension of discursive thinking as "non-discursive stability" (2009, p. 21).

- **Compassion:** the sincere aspiration for other beings to be free from suffering.

- **Loving Kindness (*metta*):** the sincere aspiration for other beings to be happy.

- **Direct Yogic Perception (of emptiness):** the direct, intuitive experience of the selfless, interconnected and interdependent nature of all phenomena, as well as, of the personal sense of self. Reality is experienced as a seamless continuum and manifestation of process.

The systematic cultivation of these wholesome mental factors is understood by many Buddhist teachers to pave the way for the eventual awakening to ultimate enlightenment. Taken together, the integration of these mental factors are the fundamental constituents of wisdom. This being said, as with all meditative practices it is critical to proceed with great care and ideally with the aid of a qualified Buddhist teacher or APT therapist.

Developing Calm Abiding

When I first began experimenting with suspending my internal dialogue as a teenager, I thought I had found the fast path to enlightenment. Of course, in reality there is no fast path to rooting out the many layers of ignorance and delusion that are the very origin of human suffering. Nonetheless, in the absence of a meditation teacher, I set out to rid myself of my ego by cutting off all discursive thinking. As it turns out, my efforts did yield some results that I have been able to refer to in the years that followed. One afternoon after practicing walking meditation for several hours and trying to cut off all discursive thinking, I arrived at my home tired and out of breath. I sat on the couch in a half lotus position and began to take notice of my breathing. As I deepened my breathing, I also focused my attention on the overhanging lamp above the dining room table. After a minute or so of this I suddenly entered a state of pure consciousness in which all sense of subjective 'self' vanished. It was as if the air between me and the lamp had become absolutely clear and focused. In point of fact, I cannot say that there was a "me" in that moment to experience anything. It was only after I came back to my ordinary mind that I was able to classify the experience at all. It would be many years before I would learn that I had a prolonged experienced No-Mind. But having had this experience I am now better predisposed, through mindfulness meditation, to have a spontaneous recognition of pure consciousness or No-Mind. Years later I would discover that what I had experienced is called the base of infinite consciousness. This is a state in which the meditator begins to perceive micro gaps in the apparent seamless continuity of self and reality.

The mental factor of calm abiding joins the ability to momentarily turn off one's discursive thinking while increasing attention to sensory input, or what Geshe Tserling refers to as "vivid intensity" (2009, p. 21). This meditative practice is essential to going into deeper levels of insight in that it provides a stable foundation of consciousness. The temporary suspending of discursive thinking is not new to Buddhism and is referred to as *mouna* in yogic meditative practices. "Mouna is a yoga practice that involves voluntary silence. You start by not speaking for a specific length of time. Mouna begins with physical silence, then blossoms into a state of total mental quietude" (Saradananda, 2011, p.39). The ultimate goal of calm abiding is just this, to *abide* with any thought, object, feeling, or sensation in a state of active witnessing. There is no pushing away of resistance; nor is there grasping at mindfulness. Rather, in calm abiding there is active acceptance of any mind state without judgment. It should also be noted that the state of mental silence is only temporary and is intended to put a check on mindless rumination and counter-productive thinking. For beginners five to ten seconds is recommended. Over time and with practice, mouna can be extended to several minutes or even an hour as in the case of advanced practitioners. However, for the purposes of entering quickly into mindful acceptance, all that is necessary is to suspend discursive thinking for a few seconds.

When learning to suspend one's internal dialogue it is best to find a quiet place that is free from distractions. It is also helpful to sit cross legged on a mat if possible, a few feet from a blank wall, and with eyes open. However, if this position is not practical, then sitting on the edge of a chair will work as well. The main idea is to sit upright without leaning on a backrest for support. This upright and unsupported posture increases alertness and focus. It also has the effect of developing one's sense of autonomy in that our sitting depends only on our own efforts. In the case of physical disability or injury it is helpful to rest the back against a chair or wall for extra support. Our gaze should be soft to take in the periphery of our vision. Our breathing is through the nose.

There are two approaches that can be utilized depending on temperament and circumstances. The first approach is to simply let the thinking activity of the mind settle down on its own for a minute or two. As our thinking mind begins to settle we focus our attention on the sensation of inhalation and exhalation through the nostrils. Gunaratana recommends that we limit our attention of breath to the sensation of air passing in and out of the nostrils. The reason for this is that by chasing our breath up and down the spine we only increase thought production. After a few minutes of relaxed nostril breathing, we then set our internal intention on turning off our discursive thinking process. At a certain point, when we are ready, we then cut off our thoughts through an act of internal effort. In the beginning the experience may only last a few seconds at a time. However, we should not become discouraged. When the thinking mind resumes, as it always will, then we simply cut off the flow of discursive thinking again. This back and forth between thinking and not thinking will go on throughout the meditation exercise. It is also useful to mentally count our in-breaths up to five times should we become too distracted. Throughout this meditative exercise we should also remember to pay close attention to all of our sensations. It is not enough to become proficient at thought-stopping to achieve calm abiding. In order to cultivate the state of calm abiding the five senses must be fully engaged as well. Engaging the five senses promotes vivid intensity.

The second method is more direct. In this approach we cut off each thought as it enters our mind. There is no letting the mind settle on its own. We simply return to the present moment while cutting off the thought process. In truth, both methods require us to, at some point, let go of our attachment to our thinking process. This is why it is best to set a specific period of time to cultivate calm abiding. Later, as we master this ability, we will be able to cut off discursive thinking at any time. However, in the beginning establishing a short and specific period of time is best. Having completed the exercise, it is good to engage in some activity to help us transition back into ordinary thinking. In time and with training, we can begin to experiment with thought stopping while engaged in everyday activity. However, in the beginning short periods of thought suspension are recommended.

Calm abiding combines non-discursive awareness *and* vivid intensity. One reason for this is that the mental state of calm abiding is an active one. We should not mistake internal stillness with being in a catatonic trance. With time and practice we can extend the state of calm abiding to fill a thirty-minute session. We can even begin to shift into calm abiding throughout the course of our busy day. We need not fear being unable to resume the ordinary flow of endless thoughts and daydreams. The brain is designed to be a thinking organ. However, in the beginning it is best to commit only short periods of time to this practice. As with all meditation, the challenge of teaching the mind to behave in unfamiliar ways can bring up past memories and impressions from the unconscious mind. This can result in emotional dysregulation in some individuals. Should the practitioner experience feelings of anger, fear, or sadness, it is wise to back off the training. Resuming the practice should only begin after the unconscious material has been understood and integrated. In extreme cases it may be necessary to cease altogether and continue the cultivation of calm abiding with the support of an experienced meditation teacher. This being said, through the practice of calm abiding we can learn to transition into more profound states of awareness. In this sense calm abiding is a little like shifting gears in a car. We must first shift into a neutral gear before shifting into a higher gear. And as always, the end objective is to empower us to greater happiness, equanimity, and freedom from suffering.

Developing Compassion and Loving Kindness

As a therapist I find it helpful to assist clients in discovering their personal recognition of their own innate goodness or Buddha Nature. I often use the metaphor of the light and tattered lampshade to illustrate the point. We all come into this life as infants who act, principally, on the inherent impulse of self-protection, the impulse to connect with others, and the impulse to express our needs and desires. I call these impulses the instinct to *connect, protect, and express*. Some will argue that we also come into a given lifetime with karmic seeds or latent behavioral tendencies (*samskaras*). However, for the purposes of the therapeutic application of Buddhism, I prefer to set aside such questions to focus on that which we can support through scientific investigation. Human beings are social animals. Like all other social animals our survival depends on the support of others of our kind. This is especially true of children and infants who lack the ability to fend for themselves. Likewise, most living creatures are impelled by the forces of DNA to avoid pain and death and to protect their offspring from harm. The human animal is no exception. For this reason we cannot be said to arrive in this life as blank slates waiting to be programmed by society to be useful members of our communities. We already possess the positive qualities of protection and connection. It is important to note that the impulse to protect is not the same as the delusion-based reaction of attacking a supposed enemy. Nor is the impulse to connect the same as taking possession of another person in an effort to control them. The impulses to connect and protect only deteriorates into attack and control when the ego function kicks in to defend the false sense of Object-Self. However, from the Process-Self perspective, there is only the spontaneous manifestation of loving protection and unity.

Returning to the light and lampshade metaphor, the light can be equated to our natural mind with its twin impulses to connect and protect. The tattered lampshade is the delusional, ego orientated mind. From the standpoint of the lampshade, the world is a threatening place filled with people with whom we feel we must compete. This is the mind of duality and fear-based, Object-Self thinking. However, no matter how dirty and tattered the lampshade becomes, the light beneath it is still pure and positive. One of the first objectives of the APT therapist is to assist the client to understand that we always have the pure light of the natural mind at our disposal.

A powerful way to deepen this understanding is to look at our own positive intentions for self-protection and connection. It is through this investigation of the impulses to connect and protect that we discover our innate reservoir of compassion and loving kindness.

Even before we begin to focus our minds in meditation, we should set our internal intention on loving kindness and compassion. There are many ways to do this depending on the individual; but no matter the method, it is our aspiration that sets the tone for the session. I like to set my aspiration on freeing all living beings from suffering and empowering them to be happy. I take a moment to imagine all people, especially those people who have wronged me in some way, as being happy and fully enlightened. I imagine what an amazing world it would be if all human beings were enlightened. I then let this mental image or object melt into pure energy that pours into my heart center. From the heart center I breathe the energy of loving kindness and compassion into my entire body. I let the space surrounding my body radiate, like the warm glow of a candle, with the energy of loving kindness and compassion. Finally, I vow to let all living beings in the universe enter into final liberation from suffering – even before myself. Of course, this is only an ideal and not a practical reality. But by making this vow I set my internal karma to compassion and loving kindness. Only then do I proceed to the next phase of my meditation to cultivate the mental factors of calm abiding.

There are many methods of developing the mental factors of compassion and loving kindness. Saint Theresa of Lisieux, The Little Flower, recommended the way of loving attention. Theresa would do everything with great attention and love to develop a spirit of gratitude and compassion. From the standpoint of APT, Theresa was combining the skills of gratitude and mindfulness to generate the mental factors of compassion and loving kindness. The skillful use of gratitude can be one of the most direct methods of connecting to our loving, natural mind or Buddha Nature. By reflecting on all that we have to be thankful for, especially when we are flooded with toxic emotions, we can come into a recognition of our natural mind. When we combine the skill of gratitude with other mindfulness skills, our experience of compassion and loving kindness is magnified significantly.

Forgiveness is another skill that we can use to develop the mental factors of compassion and loving kindness. Forgiveness is one of the most challenging skills to cultivate and one of the most important.

When we feel harmed by the actions of another trust is damaged. In some cases trust can be broken beyond repair. And in truth, there may be individuals whom we are wise to mistrust. Such people are so deluded as to be a threat to others and to themselves. But in most cases forgiveness can be achieved – if only from our side. One of the simplest methods for achieving forgiveness is to separate the behavior from the person. The old adage, hate the sin and love the sinner, comes to mind. Another method is to reflect on the suffering that is driving the harmful behavior. If the suffering – which is rooted in delusion – is removed, then the harmful behavior is likely to cease as well. It is also important to reflect on our own suffering and delusion, along with our desire to be happy and free from suffering. One of the most important people to forgive and to be grateful for is ourselves. In my work as a therapist I often see self-hatred and self-condemnation driving feelings of depression and anger. These toxic feelings then get projected onto everyone and everything around us to create a personal hell on earth. For this reason, it is always best to start with those aspects of ourselves that need forgiveness and gratitude.

Direct Perception of Emptiness

A few years following my experience of No-Mind, I was once again engaged in the daily practice of intense mindfulness meditation. I was nineteen years old and had recently returned from living in Eugene, Oregon. At the time I was mending a broken heart and was completely at loose ends with regards to my future. I took up residence at my boyhood home in Stockton, California and attempted to "get my life together". To this end I immersed myself in the study of a variety of religions, philosophies, and psychological schools of thought. Having no income and little inclination to seek work, I set out to escape the world by forcing myself into a state of higher consciousness. I took up the practice of Hath Yoga by signing up for a yoga class at the local junior college. Being that I was dependent on the somewhat unreliable system of buses in Stockton, California, I often opted to walk the ten miles to my yoga class – twenty miles if you include the return trip! Needless to say, I was in top physical form and completely drug and alcohol free. My full-time occupation was the practice of meditation.

After a period of almost nine months of daily yoga and meditation practice I was no closer to enlightenment than before. A few years had passed since my prior experience of No-Mind; but except for a few moments of relative inner stillness, I had little to show for my efforts. One evening, after returning from walking and meditating for the better part of the day, I decided to simply let my mind go and relax from my meditation practice. After running the water for a hot bath I proceeded to climb into the tub. And it was just then, as I looked down into the bath water, that I saw the clearly defined image of a human iris and pupil in the middle of my field of vision. I pulled back from the tub and ran to the mirror. As I looked at my own reflection I could also see, superimposed over my reflected image, the ghostly image of a human iris and pupil calmly staring back at me. I instantly realized that I was "seeing" my third eye or brow chakra, also referred to as *ajna* in Sanskrit. I felt a rush of panic at the possibility of losing my sanity. I imagined being overwhelmed with visions and supernatural abilities beyond my control. In an effort to calm myself, I climbed into the bath water and closed my eyes. But the image of the eye continued to stare back at me. In the days to come it would persist, regarding me with an impassionate stare; yet, for all of my fears nothing happened beyond the ordinary. I had no visions of past lives or future events. I experienced no feelings of bliss or otherworldly transcendence. My mind persisted to churn out endless thoughts and daydreams. My emotions continued to ebb and flow as usual. To this day the image of the iris and pupil rests in the middle of my field of vision. Sometimes it changes color or becomes more pronounced with regard to its intensity. However, it has never provided me with supernatural powers or abilities. It would be many years later that I would come to understand the true significance of the third eye. With the help of a psychologist who specialized in the practice of positive psychology, I was able to understand that the appearance of the third eye denotes a degree of mental stability. Furthermore, she told me, the cultivation of mental stability is critical to the direct experience of higher levels of awareness. We discussed the ramifications of awakening the brow chakra in terms of gaining clairvoyant abilities. She was quick to point out the dangers of seeking such powers for their own sake. The pursuit of psychic powers, she warned, can be an ego trip that leads to a dangerous state of self-importance.

Through my own research I would come to understand that the *ajna* center is the locus of mindful acceptance or non-grasping. In the words of yoga and meditation teacher Layne Redmond, it is at the level of *ajna* that we can experience information from the lower chakras in a state of peaceful non-attachment. "We perceive the reality of the moment rather than our habitual thoughts about reality" (2004, p. 24). From the Western medical perspective, *ajna* corresponds to a region of the brain called the anterior cingulate cortex or ACC. The ACC rests atop the limbic, emotional brain and acts to modulate the emotional impulses as they pass into the higher neocortex. As a brain structure, the ACC is most responsible for the psychological state of non-attachment. "Strengthening the ACC – such as through meditation – helps you to think clearly when you're upset, and brings warmth and emotional intelligence to your logical reasoning" (Hanson & Mendius, 2009, p. 101). The true goal of awakening the *ajna* center is to achieve the intuitive experience of ultimate reality; or what Buddhist teachers would define as emptiness. It is also the center from which arises the feeling of *pita* or spiritual joy. This being stated, it is not necessary to actually see an image of the third eye to gain the experience of emptiness and *pita*. Rather, it is enough to practice calm abiding and one-pointed mindfulness to awaken the *ajna* center. There are other meditative practices that can also prove helpful such as yogic breath work and visualizing mental objects. However, the important thing is making a strong and persistent effort.

Meditation on Emptiness

1. As before, find a quiet place to sit. We begin, as always, by setting our intention to attaining enlightenment. We then cultivate the aspiration for all living beings to be free of suffering and to be happy and at peace. Finally, we vow to hold the door open for all beings to enter into final liberation from suffering, even before ourselves.

2. The meditation begins with thinking and reflecting on the interdependent and interrelated nature of the self and phenomenon. We consider how no one thing can exist as a separate and independent entity. Rather, we understand that all things have the nature of inter-beingness. We see that self and phenomenon are co-created and re-created from one moment to the next. We then examine our own self-nature. We understand that there is no fixed

place in our mind-body complex in which we can pin down a fixed Object-Self. We reflect that all human beings go through their day with the unconscious assumption that they, alone in their uniqueness, are at the center of all existence. Finally, we reflect on the nature of emptiness and see that it is not devoid of actuality; but rather, it is filled with vast potential – dynamic, formless, and in constant process.

3. We proceed to non-attachment of body, mind, and feelings. We allow our thoughts to settle into a state of calm abiding that is free from discursive thinking. We enter into stillness and listen with the deeper mind to the vastness of the Void; of Buddha Nature. In so doing we enter into the Process-Self perspective.

4. We end the meditation by slowly returning to discursive thinking while checking into our physical bodies. It is also a good idea to begin and end any meditation session with a formal gesture such as the ringing of a ceremonial bell or bowing to one's own higher nature or power. We may reaffirm our desire that all living beings be free of suffering and to be happy and at peace. The act of bowing to the image of a sacred image is a way to promote a recognition of Buddha Nature or the natural mind.

Combining the Mental Factors of Enlightenment in Everyday Life

Taken together, the cultivation of the mental factors of calm abiding, compassion, loving kindness, and direct perception of emptiness are essential elements of the Process-Self perspective. It is not possible to force ourselves to be happy. But through the cultivation of calm abiding, compassion, loving kindness, and the direct perception of emptiness, we can begin to attune our minds and nervous systems to bliss. In his book, Eight Mindful Steps to Happiness, Bhante Gunarantana outlines the levels of psychological attainment or *jhanas* that a student must work through on the path to enlightenment. Gunarantana describes the levels of attainment as being predicated upon the development of concentration and understanding. In the first four levels the practitioner experiences feelings of joy and bliss as the nervous system becomes attuned by the practice of mindful concentration. "In the second jhana there is no more thinking to disturb the mind and disrupt its one-pointed focus. The factors of the jhana that remain are a stronger one-pointed focus of the mind, joy and happiness" (Gunarantana, 2001, p. 234). This being said, we must not let ourselves become attached to the state of bliss. To do so is to set us on a path to addiction and ego regression. Rather, when we attain to the state of ongoing bliss we must then set our sights on perfect equanimity. It is this state of being that leads to the final cessation of suffering and the awakening to abiding inner peace. The state of abiding inner peace is understood by Buddhist teachers to be the realm of Nirvana.

In my own practice of mindfulness meditation I often arrive at transitory states of bliss and equanimity. And like so many before me, I have at times sought to make bliss the goal of my efforts. Needless to say, I encountered many setbacks along the way due to grasping after bliss and inner peace. It would be years of trial and error before I would come to understand the simple truth – that inner peace is innate to who we are. What is required, through a process taking many years and ceaseless right effort, is a profound shift in perspective. And it is this shift in perspective – from the worries and self-focused concerns of the Object-Self to a free flowing and adaptive Process-Self – that sets us on a course for happiness, inner peace, and even enlightenment. It is this objective that Auto Process Therapy sets its sights upon. In the words of Buddhist meditation master Thich Nhat Hanh, "Nirvana is our true nature. Just as a wave has always been water, we have always been nirvana" (2006, 241).

Conclusion
The Future of Auto Process Therapy

"Buddhism is not a religion but a science of mind"
— Tenzin Gyatso, The 14th Dalai Lama

Although APT is in its infancy as a therapeutic modality, the validity of APT's root premise is founded upon the profound insight of Siddhartha Gautama (Gautama Buddha). It was from the Buddha's insight into the process nature of the self and reality that he devised the Four Noble Truths and the Noble Eightfold Path. APT, as a treatment model, is firmly established in Buddhism's Four Noble Truths. Whereas it is accurate to assert that Buddhism in its entirety cannot be reduced to a psychotherapeutic practice, the direct translation of Buddhist psychology into a psychotherapeutic modality is both possible and timely. In the words of Tibetan Buddhist meditation master Chogyam Trungpa, "Buddhism will come to the West as psychology" (Goleman et el., 2003, p. 72). One compelling reason for this is that Buddhism speaks directly to the issue of grasping or addiction.

Without a doubt, life in the Western world is plagued with the devastating effects of drug and alcohol abuse on family and community. With regard to alcohol addiction alone, the Diagnostic and Statistical Manual of Mental Disorders-V reports that in 2010, "44% of 12-grade students admitted to having been 'drunk in the past year', with more that 70% of college students reporting the same" (American Psychiatric Association., 2013, p. 499). Grasping or addictive behavior is one of the central areas of personal and social dysregulation that APT is designed to address.

Yet another advantage of a Buddhist psychotherapy is Buddhism's focus on the cultivation of *bodhichitta* or universal compassion in the face of anger and aggression. In our productivity driven culture we continually find ourselves in competition with everyone around us. This dog-eat-dog mindset gives rise to feelings of anger and aggression that can escalate into destructive acts. Such acts often manifest both outwardly and inwardly in destructive ways. In terms of psychotherapy anger and aggression manifest as resistance to the application of therapy. Resistance, then, presents one of the greatest stumbling blocks to successful outcomes in psychotherapy.

Lastly, Buddhism takes an unflinching stance on ignorance and denial by beginning with the truth of suffering. It is in the truth of suffering that we face the inescapable fact of impermanence and emptiness. Buddhism asserts that our denial of these facts becomes a setup for disappointment and dissatisfaction. Sadly, it is all too common for people to react to disappointment and dissatisfaction with destructive coping strategies. Such maladaptive coping strategies include using addictive substances and indulging in reckless, or even dangerous, pastimes. All of which is rooted in addiction, resistance, and denial. More than any other, these factors taken together – addiction, resistance, and denial – generate a trifecta of suffering that propels many people into emotional hell.

Without a doubt, the practice of Buddhism in the United States has taken a turn away from a formal, community-based model found within "ethnic" populations, such as the Asian or East Indian, to a more eclectic, stay-at-home and personalized Buddhist model. This shift in how Buddhism is practiced has raised much controversy between ethnic and non-ethnic practitioners. "Regarding Buddhism in the United States, there is controversy between ethnic Buddhists and Buddhists of non-Asian descent concerning how to 'practice' the religion" (Egi, 2010, p. 2). With the emergence of so many new Western psychotherapies that include Buddhist thinking and practices, this controversy will most likely increase. Furthermore, nowhere in the psychiatric community is the concept of no-abiding 'self' considered as being either possible, or desirable, as a central goal of therapy. Some within the mental health profession will, no doubt, adamantly oppose such a goal as being dangerous and impractical.

To condense the whole of Buddhism into a psychotherapeutic modality is impossible. Buddhism is a blanket term that covers a variety of study areas, some of which include ethics and morality, religious rites and rituals, meditative practices, and Buddhist psychology. APT is concerned primarily with the therapeutic application of Buddhist psychology. Therefore, if APT is to make significant inroads as a Buddhist psychotherapeutic modality, then it must remain true to Buddhism's firmly established premise of selflessness. Without adhering to the essential premise of selflessness, a Buddhist psychotherapy will remain only a cognitive-behavioral or existential model. Such a model may borrow from Buddhist thinking and practice without rising to the level of a genuine form of Buddhist psychotherapy.

The future of Auto Process Therapy will be shaped by the establishment of The Maitreya Institute of Buddhist Psychology and Auto Process Therapy. "Our problems today are no longer as simple as those encountered by the Buddha. In the twenty-first century we will have to practice meditation collectively – as a family, a city, a nation, and a community of nations. Maitreya, the Buddha of Love, may well be a community rather than an individual" (Hanh, p. 167, 1998). It will be the primary goal of the Maitreya Institute to prove and refine the efficacy of APT as an evidenced-based theory of psychotherapy. In addition, such an institute will apply the Western, scientific model of psychology to the Eastern Buddhist psychological theories already in existence. The ultimate objective of the APT Institute will be to develop an evidence-based therapeutic path to enlightenment, as defined in Buddhism, as the final cessation of suffering and the attainment of inner peace. This mind, as described by Buddhist meditation teacher and scholar Geshe Tashi Tserling in his book, The Four Noble Truths, has the characteristics of altruism and wisdom that is also beyond suffering. "The mind that realizes emptiness directly and is full of compassion – in other words the mind of bodhichitta – is the base that becomes the truth body of the Buddha" (Tserling, 2006, p. 116).

Rigorous testing and research will be required to transition Auto Process Therapy from a start-up modality to an evidence-based practice. Nonetheless, because Auto Process Therapy is grounded in the practical application of Buddhism's Four Noble Truths, APT is well positioned to make a significant contribution to the quality of mental health in Western society. Chief among these contributions are the goals of empowering clients to a greater degree of inner peace and the moment-to-moment extinction of suffering. It is to this ultimate end that Auto Process Therapy is dedicated.

Glossary of Buddhist and Auto Process Therapy Terms

Accelerated Emotional Integration (AEI): Employing mindfulness and acceptance of challenging emotions in order to return the mind to a neutral state.

Emotional Refinement: A method of rapidly refining base emotions into their more refined and adaptive states, i.e. anger into determination, fear into awareness, sadness into compassion.

Auto: Self.

Bodichitta: A Sanskrit term meaning "wise heart-mind." Referring to the Compassion/Emotional Regulation module of the APT behavioral coping skills diary card.

Buddha: A fully awakened human being. Also used to refer to Gautama Buddha, born prince Siddhartha Gautama, the historical founder of Buddhism (B.C.A. 536).

Buddhism: A spiritual and ethical wisdom path designed to extinguish suffering and lead to enlightenment.

Detachment: A temporary state of psychological separation form mental factors.

Enlightenment: A state of being fully awake to the ultimate nature of self and reality and having the characteristics of deep calm and clarity.

Fetter: An attachment to an underlying false belief that gives rise to mental anguish and delusion. There are ten fetters according to Buddhism.

Hindrance: Maladaptive states of mind defined in Buddhism as: Greed, Ill-will, Dullness and drowsiness, Restlessness or worry, and Doubt. From the point of view of APT these pathological mind states can be understood as addiction (greed), resistance (ill-will), denial (dullness), anxiety (restlessness), and depression (doubt).

Karma: Cause and effect expanding multi-directionally to produce other causes and effects and analogous to ripples in a pond. All karma is driven by choice or volition.

Maneuver: A method of guiding a client by aligning with the client's goals and intentions for therapy, as opposed to a technique or control strategy.

Mindfulness: Non-judgmental, objective awareness in-the-moment that is global and all-inclusive in nature.

Non-Attachment: The moment-to-moment letting go of mental objects, thoughts, feelings, and perceptions as they arise in the mind.

Object: A mental construct that is seen to be fixed, unchanging, and solid and that serves to ground the energies of the psyche.

Object-Self: A perspective on one's self as being fixed and permanent and likened to a solid object that travels from past to future.

Prajna: A Sanskrit or Pali word meaning "discriminating wisdom"; referring to the discernment behavioral coping skills of the APT diary card.

Process Focus: Focusing on a series of moment-to-moment changes that are devoid of a fixed and unchanging object.

Process-Self: A perspective of one's self as having the characteristics of being mutable, adaptive, focused on the present, and unhooked from past or future.

Self: The organized self of individuality arising out of underlying causes and conditions.

Samadhi: Insight into reality leading to otherworldly peace; referring to the insight behavioral coping skills of the APT diary card.

Skanda: A Tibetan or Sanskrit word that translates literally to mean "heap"; refers to the components of the Object-Self: Consciousness or Perception, Form, Feeling, Thinking, and Behavioral Habits (samskaras).

Tanha: Sanskrit. Thirst. A strong attachment for a thing, condition, state of being, or feeling; also greed and grasping.

Za: To sit.

Zen: To be awake.

Zazen: To sit in a fully awakened state of mind.

Appendix

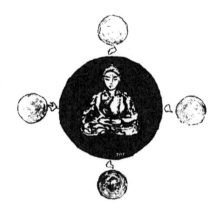

Buddhist Trifecta of Suffering

Buddha singled out three interacting dynamics that Western psychotherapists would label as addiction or greed *"lobha,"* resistance or hatred *"dosa,"* and ignorance or denial *"moha,"* as being the necessary precursors to suffering. Taken together, these three factors combine to create and sustain the trifecta of suffering or anguish.

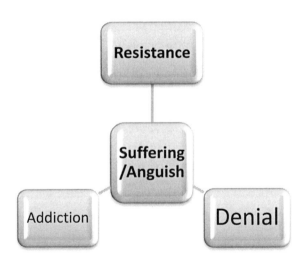

Figure 1

Buddhist Trifecta of Liberation

Liberation from the state of suffering is to be found by following a treatment program that replaces: addiction with non-attachment, resistance with unconditional acceptance, and unconsciousness with awareness, accurate understanding, and insight into the selfless nature of reality. In the Noble Eightfold Path, the Buddha outlines such a program of liberation.

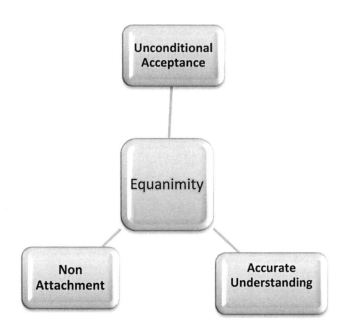

Figure 2

The Five Skandhas

The five *skandhas* are the aggregates of the Self that are generally described as being consciousness or perceptions, thoughts, form, feelings, and volition.

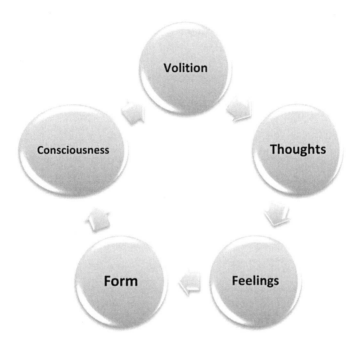

Figure 3

Working with Internal Objects

APT posits that internal objects (mental images and sounds) interact as a means of channeling the unconscious, psychic energies of aggression, desire, and anxiety. Mindfulness of the process allows us to better guide the exchange of energy to produce favorable outcomes.

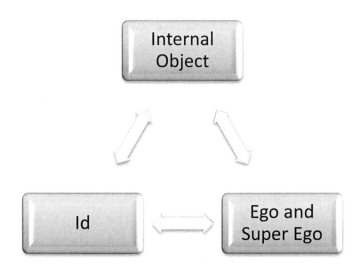

Figure 4

Behavior and Feeling

APT holds to the cognitive behavioral perspective that behavior – as defined as intentional thinking – communication, and actions interact to determine how we feel at any time.

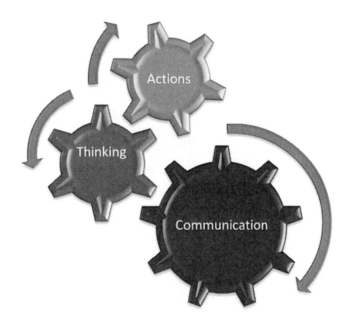

Figure 5

Object-Self versus Process-Self Perspective

Object-Self Characteristics	**Process-Self Characteristics**
1. Past and future orientation	1. Here-and-now orientation
2. Self is separate from all things (Self and others as objects to be used)	2. Self is inter-related and connected to all things (Self and others as beings to be respected)
3. Disengaged from present circumstances	3. Participates fully in the moment
4. Emotionally reactive	4. Emotionally responsive
5. Problem focused thinking	5. Solution focused thinking
6. Avoids risks	6. Acts with courage
7. Raw feelings manifest as blocked energy:	7. Raw feelings are quickly integrated and refined into constructive energy to be used:
•Anger is violence	•Anger is determination
•Fear is paralysis	•Fear is awareness
•Anxiety is agitation	•Anxiety is excitement
•Sadness is self-pity	•Sadness is compassion
•Pain is punishment	•Pain is information
•Desire is addiction	•Desire is unity
•Ignorance is denial	•Ignorance is curiosity
•Self is narcissistic projection	•Self is process
•Love is romantic delusion	•Love is truth
•Boredom is tedium	•Boredom is stability
•Grief is loss	•Grief is gratitude
8. Entrenched in habit and routine	8. Adaptive to changing circumstances
9. Attached, possessive, addiction	9. Non-attachment, able to let go
10. Resistant to change, loss, or difference	10. Unconditional acceptance of self, others, and the world
11. Denial of truth of self and circumstance	11. Actively seeks the truth of self and circumstances without fear
12. Refuses to take responsibility	12. Takes ownership

Figure 6: Object-Self versus Process-Self Perspective
The fundamental goal of Auto Process Therapy is to learn to shift the client's perspective from the Object-Self to the unfettered Process-Self perspective.

The Four Behavioral Coping Skills Modules

The four behavioral coping modules of APT differ from the Noble Eightfold Path in that they are to be learned in a non-sequential manner. This is to say, the coping behavior modules are like the petals of a flower that are connected to a central hub or core.

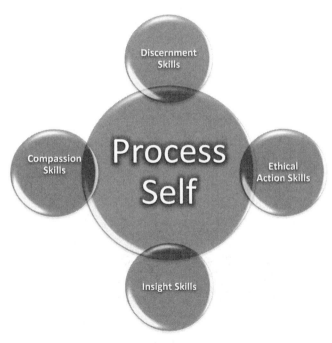

Figure 7

The Cycle of Cognition

Perceptions are information or data gathered by the five physical senses and through the sixth sense in Buddhism, the mind. The mind perceives the various cognitions that are generated within the overall field of the mind itself. Perceptions give rise to either positive or negative impulses (attraction or repulsion) that in turn prompt behaviors. Behaviors determine feelings that then influence that which we choose to perceive and how we prioritize, unconsciously, the importance of what we perceive, i.e., cognitive bias for or against.

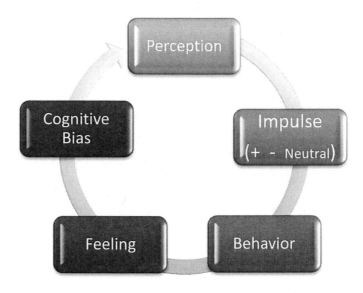

Figure 8

References

Aitken, R. (1982) Taking the path of Zen. New York: North Point Press.

American Psychiatric Association. (2013) Diagnostic and statistical manual of mental disorders. (5th ed.): Washington, DC.

Austin, J.R. (2001) Zen and the brain. Cambridge, MA. The MIT.

Press.Beck, J. (1995) Cognitive therapy: basics and beyond. New York, NY: The Guilford Press.

Beck, A., Freedma, A. (1990) Cognitive therapy of personality disorders. New York, NY: The Guilford Press.

Bhikkhu (Ed.) (2005) In the Buddha's words: An anthology of discourse from the Pali canon. Somerville, MA: Wisdom Publications, Inc.

Corey, G. (2004) Theory and Practice of group counseling. (6th ed.) Belmont, CA: Brooks/Cole-Thomson Learning.

Corsini, R., Wedding,. D., (1995). Current psychotherapies. (10th ed.) Belmont, CA: Brooks/Cole.

Csikszentmihalyi, M. (1990) Flow: The psychology of optimal experience. New York, NY: HarperCollins Publishers.

Dang. T. T. (1997) Toward the Unknown: Marital artists, what should you become? Tokyo, Japan: Charles E. Tuttle Co.

Dante. A. (2003) The Inferno. New York, NY. Barnes and Nobles Publications.

DeGraff. G. (2013). With each & every breath. Valley Center, CA. The Abbot Metta Forest Center Monastery.

Egi. L. (2010). Buddhist community: an exploration of their definition of community. Turlock, CA: California State University, Stanislaus.

Forbes. H., Post. B. (2009). Beyond logical consequences: A love based approach to helping children with survivor behaviors. Boulder, CO. Beyond Consequences Institute: LLC.

Gehart. D. (2010). Mastering competencies in family therapy. Belmont, CA: Brooks/Cole.

Galotti. K. (1999). Cognitive psychology in and out of the laboratory. (2nd ed.). Belmont, CA: Brooks/Cole.

Goleman. D. (2003). Destructive emotions: ow can we overcome them? New York, NY: Bantam Dell.

Goswami, A. (1995) The self-aware universe: how consciousness creates the material world. New York, NY: Penguin Putnam, Inc.

Gunarantana, H. (2001) Eight mindful steps to happiness: walking the Buddha's path. Somerville, MA: Wisdom Publications.

Gunarantana, H. (2011) Mindfulness in plain English. Somerville, MA: Wisdom Publications.

Gautama Buddha (1985) Exhortation to the initiates, sutra. A handbook for monks. Stockton, CA: Kinkos Copy Services.

Hanh, T. N. (1998) The Heart of the Buddha's Teaching: transforming suffering into peace, joy, and liberation. New York, NY: Broadway Books.

Hanh, T. N (2006) Understanding the mind. Berkeley, CA: Parallax Press.

Hanson, R., Mendius, R. (2009) Buddha's brain: the practical neuroscience of happiness, love, and wisdom. Oakland, CA: New Harbinger Publications.

Harris, R. (2009) ACT made simple. Oakland, CA: New Harbinger Publications.

Heinlein, R. A. (1961) Stranger in a Strange Land. New York, NY: Putnam Books.

Holiday, L. (2013) Journey to the heart of aikido: the teachings of Motomichi Anno Sensei. Berkeley, CA: Blue Snake Books.

Kraft, D. (2013) Buddha's Map: his original teachings on awakening, ease, and insight in the heart of meditation. Nevada City, CA: Blue Dolphin Publications.

Linehan, M. (1993) Cognitive behavioral treatment of borderline personality disorder. New York, NY: The Guilford Press.

Linehan, M. (1993) Skills training manual for treating borderline personality disorder. New York, NY: The Guilford Press.

Marra, T. (2005) Dialectical behavior therapy in private practice. Oakland, CA: New Harbinger Publications, Inc.

McTaggart, J. (1986) Studies in the Hegelian Dialectic. London, England: Cambridge University Press.

Metcalf, F. (2003) Buddha in your backpack. Berkeley, CA: Seastone/Ulysses Press.

Miller, W., Rollnick, S. (2002) Motivational interviewing (3rd ed.) New York, NY: The Guilford Press.

Mitchell, J. (1976) Hejira. Los Angeles, CA: A&M Studios.

Nichols, M. P., Schwartz, R. C. (2004) Family therapy: concepts and methods. (6th ed.) Person: Boston, MA.

Noss, D. (1999) A history of the world's religions (10th ed.) Prentice Hall: New Jersey, NY.

Perls, F. (1973) The gestalt approach and eyewitness to therapy. New York, NY: Random House Publishing.

Pema Chodron (2001) The places that scare you. Boston, MA. Shambhala Publications, Inc:

Redmond, L. (2004) Chakra meditation: transformation through the seven energy centers of the body. Boulder, CO: Sounds True, Inc.

Rogers, C. R. (1961) On becoming a person: a therapist's view of psychotherapy. New York, NY. Houghton Mifflin Company.

Sands, R. (1991) Clinical social work practice in community mental health. New York, NY: McMillan Publishing Company.

Sifton, E. (2005) The Serenity Prayer: faith and politics in times of peace and war. New York, NY: Norton and Company.

Tenzin Gyatso The Awakening Mind.: Somerville, MA. Wisdom Publications.

Tenzin Gyatso (2005) Essence of the heart sutra. (Thupten Jinpa, Ed.) Somerville, MA. Wisdom Publications.

Tserling, T. (2006) Buddhist Psychology: the foundations of Buddhist thought. Somerville, MA. Wisdom Publications.

Tserling, T. (2008) The Awakened Mind: The foundations of Buddhist thought. Wisdom Publications: Somerville, MA.

Tserling, T. (2009) Emptiness: the foundations of Buddhist thought. Wisdom Publications: Somerville, MA.

Obeku Shu (1982) Soto Shu Sutras (2nd ed.) Tokyo, Japan: Kinko Printing.

Uesiba, M. (1992) The art of peace. Boston, MA. Shambhala Publications, Inc.

Yalom, I. (1995) The theory and practice of group psychotherapy (4th ed.) New York, NY: Basic Books.